Intern Tips in Obstetrics and Gynecology

Disclaimer

The purpose of this book is providing a clinical decision pathway with a survey of treatment options, to accommodate the educational interests of trainees and practitioners in addressing the scope of options that might be considered in their clinical practice. There is no assurance that the scope of clinical decision-making and treatment options outlined for any particular condition and/or individual clinical presentation is comprehensive. The publisher and authors of this book disclaim any liability, loss, injury or damage incurred as a consequence, directly or indirectly, of the use and application of any of the contents of this learning material.

Intern Tips in
Obstetrics and Gynecology

Sanja Kupesic Plavsic MD PhD
Assistant Dean for Faculty Development
Professor
Department of Obstetrics and Gynecology
Paul L Foster School of Medicine
Texas Tech University Health Sciences Center
El Paso, Texas, USA

Jennifer Molokwu MD MPH
Assistant Professor
Department of Family and Community Medicine
Paul L Foster School of Medicine
Texas Tech University Health Sciences Center
El Paso, Texas, USA

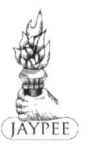

The Health Sciences Publisher

New Delhi | London | Philadelphia | Panama

Jaypee Brothers Medical Publishers (P) Ltd.

Headquarters
Jaypee Brothers Medical Publishers (P) Ltd.
4838/24, Ansari Road, Daryaganj
New Delhi 110 002, India
Phone: +91-11-43574357
Fax: +91-11-43574314
E-mail: jaypee@jaypeebrothers.com

Overseas Offices

J.P. Medical Ltd.
83, Victoria Street, London
SW1H 0HW (UK)
Phone: +44-20 3170 8910
Fax: +44(0) 20 3008 6180
E-mail: info@jpmedpub.com

Jaypee-Highlights Medical Publishers Inc.
City of Knowledge, Bld. 237, Clayton
Panama City, Panama
Phone: +1 507-301-0496
Fax: +1 507-301-0499
E-mail: cservice@jphmedical.com

Jaypee Medical Inc.
325, Chestnut Street
Suite 412, Philadelphia, PA 19106, USA
Phone: +1 267-519-9789
E-mail: support@jpmedus.com

Jaypee Brothers Medical Publishers (P) Ltd.
17/1-B, Babar Road, Block-B, Shaymali
Mohammadpur, Dhaka-1207
Bangladesh
Mobile: +08801912003485
E-mail: jaypeedhaka@gmail.com

Jaypee Brothers Medical Publishers (P) Ltd.
Bhotahity, Kathmandu, Nepal
Phone: +977-9741283608
E-mail: kathmandu@jaypeebrothers.com

Website: www.jaypeebrothers.com
Website: www.jaypeedigital.com

© 2016, Jaypee Brothers Medical Publishers

The views and opinions expressed in this book are solely those of the original contributor(s)/author(s) and do not necessarily represent those of editor(s) of the book.

All rights reserved. No part of this publication may be reproduced, stored or transmitted in any form or by any means, electronic, mechanical, photocopying, recording or otherwise, without the prior permission in writing of the publishers.

All brand names and product names used in this book are trade names, service marks, trademarks or registered trademarks of their respective owners. The publisher is not associated with any product or vendor mentioned in this book.

Medical knowledge and practice change constantly. This book is designed to provide accurate, authoritative information about the subject matter in question. However, readers are advised to check the most current information available on procedures included and check information from the manufacturer of each product to be administered, to verify the recommended dose, formula, method and duration of administration, adverse effects and contraindications. It is the responsibility of the practitioner to take all appropriate safety precautions. Neither the publisher nor the author(s)/editor(s) assume any liability for any injury and/or damage to persons or property arising from or related to use of material in this book.

This book is sold on the understanding that the publisher is not engaged in providing professional medical services. If such advice or services are required, the services of a competent medical professional should be sought.

Every effort has been made where necessary to contact holders of copyright to obtain permission to reproduce copyright material. If any have been inadvertently overlooked, the publisher will be pleased to make the necessary arrangements at the first opportunity.

Inquiries for bulk sales may be solicited at: jaypee@jaypeebrothers.com

Intern Tips in Obstetrics and Gynecology

First Edition: 2016
ISBN: 978-93-5152-478-6
Printed at Rajkamal Electric Press, Plot No. 2, Phase-IV, Kundli, Haryana.

Dedicated to

My boys Branko, Ivor and Hobbes

Sanja Kupesic Plavsic

My parents Odih and
Nwakego Molokwu

Jennifer Molokwu

Preface

Intern Tips in Obstetrics and Gynecology aims to provide physicians still in training, physicians-in-practice, midwives and medical students with a quick reference for commonly seen inpatient obstetric and gynecological issues. Some of the currently available resources do not include specific medications, dosages and interventions that are needed at the point of care. Frequently, there is not enough time to read an article through a large reference when there is a patient need that requires an immediate response. The book serves as a reference and a simple starting point to assist in making an initial decision.

The book contains the information to cover common inpatient cases seen on obstetrics and gynecology inpatient rounds. Sample orders and notes are included to help the provider and physician-in-training to focus on the points that are important to address.

The book is organized by topic and addresses wide differential diagnosis concerns and specific diagnostic work-up for common patient presentations.

The book attempts to point the clinician in the proper initial direction to assist in disposition, initial management and initial patient work-up.

Sanja Kupesic Plavsic
Jennifer Molokwu

Acknowledgments

We would like to thank all of our students and residents who challenged and pushed us ever forward. Our special thanks to Dr Lisa Montgomery who proposed and initiated this project.

We also like to thank the dedicated staff of M/s Jaypee Brothers Medical Publishers (P) Ltd, New Delhi, India, who were willing to dedicate their time and energy to this project. The team has always provided excellent technical support.

Contents

1. Normal Pregnancy   1

General Labor and Delivery Tips   *1*
Inpatient Types and Notes   *3*
Routine Prenatal Visit and Note   *4*
Specific Prenatal Visit Components   *5*
Combined Quad Test   *6*
Calculating/Estimating Gestational Age   *7*
Rhesus Alloimmunization   *9*
Information Needed in Every Obstetrics Note   *10*
Physical Examination of Pregnant Patient   *11*
Group B Streptococcus Screening   *11*
Antibiotics for Group B Streptococcus Prophylaxis   *13*
Fetal Assessment   *13*
Advanced Fetal Testing   *15*
Fetal Ultrasound Testing   *16*
Assessment of Fetal Wellbeing   *17*
Intrapartum Fetal Monitoring   *18*
Decelerations in Detail   *20*
Metabolic Changes in Pregnancy   *22*

Endocrine System Changes *23*
Steroid Changes in Pregnancy *24*
Gastrointestinal System Changes *25*
Respiratory and Cardiovascular Changes *26*
Hematologic Changes *27*
Genitourinary and Renal Changes *28*
Central Nervous System and Skin Changes in Pregnancy *29*

2. Pregnancy Complications — 37

Triage Tips *37*
Sample Triage/Labor and Delivery H+P Note *39*
Gestational Diabetes Mellitus *40*
HIV in Pregnancy *41*
Intrauterine Growth Restriction *42*
Thyroid in Pregnancy *43*
Epilepsy *44*
Abdominal and Renal Disorders *45*
Gestational Hypertension *46*
Pre-eclampsia *47*
Eclampsia *48*
Antihypertensive/Anticonvulsant Doses *48*
Hemolysis, Elevated Liver Enzymes, Low Platelets Syndrome *49*
Thrombosis *50*

Peripartum Cardiomyopathy *51*
First Trimester Bleeding *52*
Third Trimester Bleeding *53*
Ectopic Pregnancy *55*
Placenta Previa *56*
Placental Abruption *57*
Uterine Rupture *58*
Vasa Previa *58*
Fetal Demise *59*
Induced Abortion *60*
Abortion Methods *61*
Medications in Pregnancy *62*
Antibiotics, Androgens and Pain Medications *63*
Asthmatic and Cardiovascular Medications *64*

3. Labor and Delivery   72

Labor Progress, Vaginal Delivery Notes *72*
Assessing a Patient in Labor *76*
Rupture of Membranes *77*
Vaginal Examinations *78*
Digital Cervical Examination *79*
Labor Pain Control *80*
Stages of Labor *81*
Labor Movements *83*
Postpartum Note *84*

xiv Intern Tips in Obstetrics and Gynecology

4. Abnormal Labor — 88

Labor Induction *88*
Cesarean Section *89*
Preterm Labor *91*
Magnesium Note *94*
Management of Prematures Rupture of Membranes *95*
Labor Dystocia *96*
Abnormal Third Stage of Labor *97*
Postpartum Hemorrhage *98*
Shoulder Dystocia *100*
Breech *101*

5. Postpartum — 105

Immediate Postdelivery Tasks *105*
Routine Postpartum Care *106*
Discharge Planning *108*
Postpartum Maternal Changes *109*
Breastfeeding *110*
Postpartum Infections *111*
Postpartum Psychiatric Complications *112*

6. Gynecology Consult — 116

Gynecologic Clinic Note *116*
Complete Gynecologic History *117*

Procedure and Postoperative Notes *118*
Postoperative Concerns in Gynecology *119*
Uterine Bleeding *120*
Dysfunctional Uterine Bleeding *121*
Menopause *123*
Pre- and Postmenopausal Bleeding *124*
Pelvic Pain (Acute and Chronic) *125*
Pelvic Inflammatory Disease *126*
Toxic Shock Syndrome *127*
Incontinence and Pelvic Organ Prolapse *128*
Gestational Trophoblastic Disease *129*
Ovarian Cyst Management *130*
Cancer Screening Don'ts *132*
Cervical Dysplasia Classification *133*
Gynecologic Cancer *134*
Cervical Cancer FIGO Staging *135*
Endometrial Cancer FIGO Staging *136*
Ovarian Cancer FIGO Staging *137*
Vaginal and Vulvar Cancer FIGO Staging *138*

Index *145*

Abbreviations

&: And
<: Under or less than
1LTCS: Primary low transverse cesarean section
ABC: Airway breathing circulation
ABG: Arterial blood gas
ACE: Angiotensin converting enzyme
AD: Autosomal dominant
AFI: Amniotic fluid index
AFP: Alpha feto-protein
AGA: Average for gestational age
AMA: Advanced maternal age
AR: Autosomal recessive
ART, ARV: Antiretroviral therapy
BM: Bowel movement
BP: Blood pressure
BPP: Biophysical profile
BTL: Bilateral tubal ligation
BUN: Blood urea nitrogen
Ca: Calcium or cancer
CAH: Congenital adrenal hyperplasia
CBC: Complete blood count
CHD: Congenital heart disease
CHF: Congestive heart failure
Cl: Chloride
cm: Centimeter
CMV: Cytomegalovirus
CN: Cranial nerve
COPD: Chronic obstructive pulmonary disease
CPAP: Continuous positive airway pressure
Cr: Creatinine
C-section: Cesarean section
CST: Contraction stress test
CT: Computerized tomography

CXR: Chest X-ray
D+C: Dilatation and curettage
D10: 10 percent dextrose
DKA: Diabetic ketoacidosis
dL: Deciliter
DLD: Dyslipidemia
DM: Diabetes mellitus
DUB: Dysfunctional uterine bleeding
DVT: Deep vein thrombosis
EBL: Estimated blood loss
ECG/EKG: Electrocardiogram
ED: Emergency department
EDD: Estimated date of delivery
EFW: Estimated fetal weight
e.g.: For example
EP: Ectopic pregnancy
esp: Especially
etc.: Et cetera
EtOH: Alcohol, ethanol
FFP: Fresh frozen plasma
FHR: Fetal heart rate
FHT: Fetal heart tones
FM: Fetal movement
g: Gram
G: Gravidity
GA: Gestational age
GBS: Group *B Streptococcus*
GC/Chlamydia: *Neisseria gonorrhoeae* and *Chlamydia trachomatis* testing
GDM: Gestational diabetes mellitus
GFR: Glomerular filtration rate
GH: Growth hormone
GI: Gastrointestinal
GTT: Glucose tolerance test
h/o: History of
HA: Hemolytic anemia
HBV: Hepatitis B virus
hCG: Human chorionic gonadotropin
HCT: Hematocrit
HCV: Hepatitis C virus
HELLP: Hemolysis, elevated liver enzymes, low platelets
Hgb: Hemoglobin

HIV: Human immunodeficiency virus

HPI: History of present illness

HR: Heart rate

hrs: Hours

HSV: Herpes simplex virus

ICU: Intensive Care Unit

IM: Intramuscular

IUD: Intrauterine device

IUGR: Intrauterine growth restriction

IV: Intravenous

IVF: Intravenous fluid

IVP: Intravenous push

K: Potassium

kg: Kilogram

L: Liter

L&D: Labor and delivery

LFT: Liver function test

LGA: Large for gestational age

LIQORAA: Location, intensity, quality, onset, radiation, aggravating, alleviating

LMWH: Low molecular weight heparin

LOF: Loss of fluid

LR: Lactated ringers (Ringers Lactate)

LTCS: Low transverse cesarean section

Mg: Magnesium or milligram

mL: Milliliter

mm: Millimeter

mo: Month

MSAFP: Maternal serum alpha-fetoprotein

Mx: Management

MRSA: Methicillin resistant *Staphylococcus aureus*

MSSA: Methicillin-susceptible *Staphylococcus aureus*

Na: Sodium

NS: Normal saline

NST: Nonstress test

NSVD: Normal spontaneous vaginal delivery

OB GYN: Obstetrics and gynecology

OPQRST: Onset, provokes, quality, radiation, severity, timing

OTC meds: Over the counter medications

P: Parity
PE: Physical exam
PGE: Prostaglandin E2
PNV: Prenatal vitamins
PO: By mouth
PPROM: Preterm premature rupture of membranes
PRBC: Packed red blood cells
PROM: Premature rupture of membranes
PTX: Pneumothorax
pulm: Pulmonary
q: Every
r/o: Rule out
RBC: Red blood cell
RCS: Repeat cesarean section
Rh: Rhesus
ROM: Rupture of membranes
ROS: Review of systems
RPR: Rapid plasma reagin
s/s: Signs and symptoms
SBP: Systolic blood pressure
SCD: Sequential compression device
SGA: Small for gestational age
SIDS: Sudden infant death syndrome
SOB: Shortness of breath
SSE: Sterile speculum exam
SVE: Sterile vaginal exam
STD: Sexually transmitted disease
tx: Treatment
T 1,2,3: Trimester 1,2,3
UA: Urinalysis
UFH: Unfractionated heparin
UOP: Urine output
US: Ultrasound
VB: Vaginal bleeding
VBAC: Vaginal birth after cesarean
VDRL: Venereal disease research laboratory
wk: Week
wks: Weeks
yr: Year
yrs: Years
y/o: Years old

1
Normal Pregnancy

CHAPTER OUTLINES

- General Labor and Delivery Tips
- Inpatient Types and Notes
- Routine Prenatal Visit and Note
- Specific Prenatal Visit Components
- Combined Quad Test
- Calculating/Estimating Gestational Age
- Rhesus Alloimmunization
- Information Needed in Every Obstetrics Note
- Physical Examination of Pregnant Patient
- Group B *Streptococcus* Screening
- Antibiotics for Group B *Streptococcus* Prophylaxis
- Fetal Assessment
- Advanced Fetal Testing
- Fetal Ultrasound Testing
- Assessment of Fetal Wellbeing
- Intrapartum Fetal Monitoring
- Decelerations in Detail
- Metabolism Changes during Pregnancy
- Endocrine System Changes
- Steroid Changes in Pregnancy
- Gastrointestinal System Changes
- Respiratory and Cardiovascular Changes
- Hematologic Changes
- Genitourinary and Renal Changes
- Central Nervous Sysytem and Skin Changes in Pregnancy

GENERAL LABOR AND DELIVERY TIPS

- Round on your patient and learn their background and vitals. Be prepared to present your patient at snapshot/board rounds, where all the antepartum patients are discussed.

- Always remember to say why a patient had a C-section, and for postpartum plans include birth control and method of feeding (breast/bottle).
- During the day, on both short and long call, you will check on your patients, perform cervical checks and *mag* checks (routine checks on your patients who are on magnesium prophylaxis), triage patients, and deliver babies.
  - Physically be on L&D for the entirety of your call. Otherwise, you will frequently miss out on the delivery of a patient you have been following all day.
- The "board" is a list with all of the laboring patients, their diagnoses, and other pertinent information. It is usually run and updated by the third-year resident. This is where you can find out when a patient's next cervix check or *mag* check is due, whether they are delivering vaginally or by C-section, etc.
- Maternal fetal medicine (MFM) is the high-risk obstetrics service. These patients may be antepartum or postpartum. Interns typically see only the postpartum patients on this service. There are typically three types of patients on the high risk service:
  1. Patients with complications of pregnancy, e.g. premature rupture of membranes or pre-eclampsia
  2. Patients with medical problems that complicate pregnancy, e.g. lupus
  3. Healthy patients with high-risk babies, e.g. intrauterine growth restriction (IUGR)

INPATIENT TYPES AND NOTES

- Triage
  - Patient is usually first evaluated by the nurse, then the intern. Based on their presentations, the decision is made to admit, observe or discharge.
- Laboring patients
  - Need progress notes every 4 hours in latent phase and every 2 hours in active labor.
  - You should meet the patient prior to pushing. If not possible, meet all your patients as early in the shift as you can.
  - Learn to gown and glove quickly. Deliveries happen whether you are ready or not.
- Antepartum patients
  - Need progress notes every 4 hours that address the fetal wellbeing (FHT, strip), LOF, VB. If the patient is there for a maternal reason, include a maternal physical examination.
  - Typical diagnosis is premature rupture of membranes, preterm labor, placenta previa, pre-eclampsia, or medical complications of pregnancy.
- *Mag* notes are needed every 4 hours, including monitoring for magnesium toxicity
  - Respiratory depression (oxygen saturations)
  - Pulmonary edema (lung examination)
  - Renal failure (urine output)
  - Neurologic irritation (deep tendon reflexes)
  - Worsening blood pressure, signs of fetal distress
- Postpartum patients need daily progress notes.

ROUTINE PRENATAL VISIT AND NOTE

- Frequency of visits
  - Before 28 weeks gestation, patients are seen every 4 weeks.
  - Between 28 and 36 weeks gestation, patients are seen every 2 weeks.
  - After 36 weeks, patients are seen weekly.
- At each visit
  - Check patient's weight gain, urine, blood pressure, fetal heart tones and fundal height. Ask about fetal movement, vaginal bleeding, loss of fluid, contractions, vaginal discharge, dysuria, nausea/vomiting and intake of prenatal vitamins.
  - Other questions based on past medical history or complications of the pregnancy.
- Prenatal visit note
  - *Subjective:* Address FM, LOF, VB, contractions
  - *Objective:* BP, weight, urinalysis, fundal height, fetal heart rate, extremity edema.
  - A ___ y/o G__P__@ __weeks/days gestation by LMP (or other method of dating here) presents with (signs and symptoms)
    - *Prenatal labs:* Blood type Ab/HIV/Hep B/RPR NR/RNI/CF/GC/CT/Hgb/Pap/Rhogam.
    - Return visit in __ weeks.

SPECIFIC PRENATAL VISIT COMPONENTS

- Initial visit:
  - *Labs:* Complete blood cell (CBC), type and screen, antibody screen, Rubella, RPR (VDRL), HBsAg, hepatitis C virus (HCV), HIV, Pap (if due per screening guidelines), GC/Chlamydia, UA and culture, Hgb electrophoresis if African descent. Dating US if uncertain last menstrual period (LMP).
  - Initial visit counseling on diet and exercise, weight gain, over-the-counter (OTC) medicines, environmental exposure, travel, frequency of visits, ED precautions.
- Additional checks at specific visits
  - 10-12 weeks gestation—check fetal heart tone (FHT) with Doppler
  - 11-14 weeks—first trimester combined screen optional
  - 15-20 weeks—Quad screen (AFP, Estriol, Free b-hCG, inhibin).
    - Offer amniocentesis for advanced maternal age (AMA) or family history of genetic disease.
    - Ultrasound (anatomy scan) from 18 to 20 weeks
  - 21-25 weeks—fundal height in centimeter correlates with gestational age in weeks +/-2.
  - 26-28 weeks—1 hour glucose screen (50 g).
    - Rhogam injection if mother is Rh negative.
    - Sign tubal papers if patient desires BTL.
  - 35-36 weeks—GBS culture. Discuss labor signs.
  - 41+weeks—review estimated date of delivery (EDD) dating criteria. Assess Bishop's score. Consider induction.

COMBINED QUAD TEST

- First trimester combined test screens for trisomy 21 and 18 (with maternal age).
  - Between 11 and 14 weeks gestation (blood can be collected as early as 9 weeks).
  - Maternal serum pregnancy-associated plasma protein A (PAPP-A)—low in trisomy 21 and very low in trisomy 18.
  - US measurement of nuchal translucency—increased in trisomy 21 and trisomy 18.
  - Maternal serum b-hCG levels—high in trisomy 21, low in trisomy 18 and anencephaly.
  - Positive cut off values are individual to testing centers (commonly at >1 in 300). If positive, offer genetic screening with chorionic villus sampling (prior to 14 weeks).
- From 15 to 22 weeks gestation use the Quadruple test (as early as possible).
  - Maternal serum alpha-fetoprotein (MSAFP) is most accurate between 16 and 18 weeks. Inaccurate dating is the most common reason for an abnormal screen.
    - *High levels:* Neural tube defects, abdominal wall defects (gastroschisis and omphalocele); fetal death; placental abnormalities (abruption); multiple gestation.
    - *Low levels:* Seen in up to 21% of Down's syndrome fetuses (trisomy 21).
  - *Unconjugated estriol (uE3):* Low in trisomy 21, 18 and sometimes low in trisomy 13.

- *Beta-hCG:* Double normal levels in trisomy 21.
- *Inhibin A:* Can be double normal levels in trisomy 21.
- *Cell free DNA:* It can be performed starting at 9 weeks. Has a high sensitivity and specificity for trisomy 18 and trisomy 21, not as high for trisomy 13. Can be used to determine gender. Results still require confirmation with diagnostic tests.

CALCULATING/ESTIMATING GESTATIONAL AGE

- Definition of terms:
  - *Gestational age (GA):* The number of weeks of pregnancy counting from the first day of the last menstrual period (LMP).
  - *Developmental age:* Weeks counting from fertilization.
  - *Embryo:* Fertilization to 8 weeks.
  - *Fetus:* From 8 weeks until birth.
  - *Previable:* Before 24 weeks.
  - *Preterm:* 24–37 weeks.
  - *Term:* 37–42 weeks.
  - *First trimester:* 0–14 weeks.
  - *Second trimester:* 14–28 weeks.
  - *Third trimester:* 28 weeks to birth.
- Using LMP to calculate the due date:
  - *Naegele's rule:* Calculate the estimated date of confinement (due date) +/– 2 weeks.
  - First day of patient's last normal menstrual period— 3 months + 7 days + 1 year.

- Using ultrasound:
  - First trimester ultrasound accurate +/− 5 days
  - US at 13–20 weeks accurate +/− 7 days
  - US at 20+ weeks accurate +/− 21 days
- *Clinical examination:* Estimate using bimanual/fundal height (Table 1.1).

Table 1.1: Clinical examination: Estimate using bimanual/fundal height

Nongravid	8 cm (plum size)
4–6 weeks	10 cm (orange size)
8–10 weeks	12 cm (grapefruit size)
12 weeks	Top of pubic symphysis
16 weeks	Half way to umbilicus
20 weeks	At umbilicus
20–36 weeks	Height in centimeter from pubic symphysis (GA in weeks +/− 2 weeks)

- Using fetal heart tones
  - 5% Doppler tones heard by 8 weeks.
  - 95% Doppler tones heard by 12 weeks.
- *Using quickening:* Sensation of movement felt on 3 consecutive days (multiparous patients usually between 16–18 weeks; primiparous patients usually between 18–20 weeks).

RHESUS ALLOIMMUNIZATION

- If the pregnant female is Rh− and her fetus is Rh+, she may become sensitized to the Rh antigen and develop antibodies. These antibodies may cross the placenta and attack the fetal RBCs and cause fetal RBC hemolysis.
- Sensitization may occur during:
  - Amniocentesis, miscarriage/threatened abortion, vaginal bleeding, placental abruption/previa, delivery, abdominal trauma, cesarean section, external version.
- Sensitization can cause fetal danger (when a mom is exposed to Rh+ blood she develops antibodies; in a later pregnancy, her immune system that already recognizes Rh+ blood, crosses the placenta and attacks Rh+ fetal blood).
- *Screening:* Determine maternal Rh type and measure antibody at the initial visit with an indirect Coombs' test.
- *Rhogam:* IgG that will attach to the Rh antigen and prevent immune response.
  - *Rh−mom with a negative initial antibody screen (at 0, and 24-28 weeks):* Give 300 µg Rh IgG to prevent antibody formation. At birth, if baby is Rh+ give postpartum Rh IgG.
  - *Rh−mom with an initial positive antibody screen at 0 and 12-20 weeks:* Check the antibody titer. If titer remains < 1:16, the risk of hemolytic disease of the newborn is low. If the titer is > 1:16 or rising, the likelihood of hemolytic disease of the newborn is high. Amniocentesis begins at 16-20 weeks gestational age to analyze fetal cells for Rh status.

INFORMATION NEEDED IN EVERY OBSTETRICS NOTE

- OB history
  - *G (gravidity):* Total number of pregnancies, including normal and abnormal intrauterine pregnancies, abortions, ectopic pregnancies, and hydatidiform moles (remember, if patient was pregnant with twins, G =1).
  - *P (parity):* Number of deliveries > 500 g or ≥24 weeks' gestation, stillborn (dead) or alive (if patient was pregnant with twins, P = 1).
    - T = number of term deliveries
    - P = number of preterm deliveries
    - A = number of abortions
    - L = number of living children
- Delivery history
  - History of patient's prior pregnancies, with outcome of each (NSVD, C/S, D&C, etc.). Relate weeks of gestation, gender, mode of delivery, weight of infant, complications during pregnancy and delivery, etc.
- History of current pregnancy/HPI
  - *EGA:* Estimated gestational age
  - *EDC:* Estimated date of confinement, by LMP or by US
  - Where was the prenatal care, how many visits, when was the last visit
  - List the labs and results
  - Ask about vaginal bleeding/contractions/fetal movement/loss of water

Normal Pregnancy

PHYSICAL EXAMINATION OF PREGNANT PATIENT

- *Abdomen:* Gravid, tenderness?
- *EFW:* Estimated fetal weight by Leopold's
- Presentation
- Placental location, AFI (confirm by US)
- Adequate pelvis?
- *VE:* Vaginal examination—dilatation/% effacement/station
- *SSE:* Sterile speculum exam (Nitrazine? Pooling? Ferning? Membranes intact?)
- *Fetal monitoring:* Baseline heart rate, reactive?
- *Toco:* How frequent are contractions?
- *Beta hCG:* Use urine levels to diagnose pregnancy.
  - Use quantitative serum in evaluating for ectopic pregnancy, monitoring trophoblastic tumors, screening for fetal anomalies.
  - Beta hCG levels from weeks 4 to 8 should double every 48-72 hours—the alpha subunit of hCG is identical to the alpha subunit of LH, FSH and TSH.
- Doppler fetal heart tones are heard by 8 weeks. If not heard by 11 weeks, evaluate for a viable intrauterine pregnancy by ultrasound.
- *Fundal height:* 16 weeks, midway between pubis and umbilicus. 20 weeks at umbilicus (*See* Table 1.1).

GROUP B STREPTOCOCCUS SCREENING

- All women are to have a GBS (group B *Streptococcus*) culture at 35-37 weeks to determine need for GBS prophylaxis during labor.

- Prophylaxis is not indicated for previous pregnancy with positive screen (planned C-section without onset of labor or rupture of membranes), and current pregnancy negative screen (negative GBS screen requires no prophylaxis regardless of intrapartum risk factors).
- No GBS screen required and automatic antibiotic prophylaxis if a woman has had GBS bacteria during the current pregnancy or a previous infant with invasive GBS disease.
- Antibiotic prophylaxis if unknown GBS status and a risk factor such as:
    - Delivery under 37 weeks gestation
    - Ruptured membranes for longer than 18 hours during labor
    - Intrapartum fever over 38°C unless amnionitis is suspected, then give a broad-spectrum antibiotic therapy, instead of prophylaxis

- GBS prophylaxis is also given to women <37 weeks gestation with:
    - Onset of labor or rupture of membranes and risk for preterm delivery, and unknown GBS.
    - Order antibiotics for at least 48 hours, unless delivery occurs sooner (may be continued beyond 48 hours in a GBS culture positive woman if delivery has not occurred). For women who are GBS culture positive, antibiotics should be reinitiated when labor likely to proceed to delivery occurs.

- If no delivery within 4 weeks, a vaginal and rectal GBS screening culture should be repeated and the patient managed based on the result of the repeat culture.

ANTIBIOTICS FOR GROUP B STREPTOCOCCUS PROPHYLAXIS

- *Preferred:* Penicillin G 5 million units IV × 1 dose, then 2.5 million units IV q4h until delivery.
- *Alternative:* Ampicillin 2 g IV × 1 dose, then 1 g IV q4h until delivery.
- If patient is Penicillin-allergic
  - *If low-risk for anaphylaxis:* Cefazolin 2 g IV × 1 dose then 1 g IV q8h until delivery
  - *If high-risk for anaphylaxis:* Past anaphylaxis with Penicillin or history of asthma or beta blocker use:
    - Determine GBS susceptibility to Clindamycin and Erythromycin
    - *If susceptible give:* Clindamycin 900 mg IV q8h until delivery or Erythromycin 500 mg IV q6h until delivery.
- If GBS resistant to Clindamycin and Erythromycin or susceptibility unknown give Vancomycin 1g IV q12h until delivery (reserved for Penicillin-allergic women at high-risk for anaphylaxis).

FETAL ASSESSMENT

- Leopold maneuvers assess the fetus and maternal abdomen
  - *First:* Feel the top of the uterus—"What fetal part occupies the fundus?"

- *Second:* Feel sides of uterus—"On what side is the fetal back?"
- *Third:* Place thumb on one side of the lower uterine segment and the first finger on the other—"What fetal part lies over the pelvic inlet?"
- *Fourth:* Face the patient's feet and place both hands on both sides of her uterus—"On which side is the cephalic prominence?"

- Station is the degree of descent of the presenting part in relation to ischial spines.
  - The ischial spine is zero station and the areas above and below are divided into thirds.
  - Above the ischial spines are stations −3, −2, and −1, with −1 being closest to the spines.
  - Positive stations are below the ischial spines. +3 station is the level of the introitus.
- *Lie describes the relation of the long-axis of the fetus to that of the mother:* longitudinal (99%), transverse or oblique.
- Presentation is the fetal part at the cervix.
- Normal is a cephalic presentation with posterior fontanel as the presenting part (vertex).
- If the lie is transverse, the shoulder is the presenting part.
- Longitudinal will present with either the head (cephalic) or buttocks (breech).
- *Position is the relation to the maternal pelvis:* Facing the right (R) or left (L) side, presenting part (occiput, sacrum or mentum) and its direction anteriorly (A), transversely (T), or posteriorly (P).
- *Attitude:* Flexed or extended.

Normal Pregnancy

ADVANCED FETAL TESTING

- Amniocentesis is performed at 15 weeks GA when the amniotic fluid volume is approximately 200 mL.
    - *Indications:* Fetal anomaly suspected on US, abnormal MSAFP, family history of congenital abnormalities, offered to all patients ≥ 35 years of age.
    - *Procedure:* Amniotic fluid is aspirated with ultrasound guidance. AFP levels are performed on the extracted fluid and fetal cells can be grown for karyotyping or DNA assays.
    - *Risks:* Pain/cramping, vaginal spotting/amniotic fluid leakage in 1–2% of cases, symptomatic amnionitis in < 1/1,000 patients, rate of fetal loss ≤ 0.5%.
- *Chorionic villus sampling (CVS).* A sample of villi is taken and analyzed.
    - Between 9 and 12 weeks GA. Allows for chromosomal status, fetal karyotyping, and biochemical assays or DNA tests to be done earlier than amniocentesis.
    - *Risks:* Preterm delivery, premature rupture of membranes, fetal injury.
- *Cordocentesis:* A spinal needle is advanced under US guidance into a cord vessel to sample fetal blood.
    - Genetic testing, performed after 17 weeks.
    - *Indications:* Fetal karyotyping, to determine the fetal hematocrit in Rh isoimmunization, assay fetal platelet counts, acid–base status, antibody levels, blood chemistries, etc.

- *FISH (fluorescent in situ hybridization):* A specific DNA probe with a fluorescent label that binds homologous DNA → allows identification of specific sites.
    - *Karyotyping:* Visualize chromosome size, banding pattern, and centromere position.
    - *Indications:* Advanced maternal age, previous child with abnormal karyotype, parental chromosome rearrangements, fetal structural abnormality on sonogram, unexplained intrauterine growth restriction (IUGR), abnormally low MSAFP.

FETAL ULTRASOUND TESTING

- Ultrasound is used to:
    - Confirm an intrauterine pregnancy
    - Find fetal heartbeats
    - Diagnose multiple gestations
    - Estimate gestational age
    - Screen for fetal structural anomalies
- Major limitation is that dating is less accurate after 20 weeks.
- *Ultrasound:* Intrauterine pregnancy seen on transvaginal US when beta hCG >1,500; seen on abdominal US when beta-hCG >6,000 mIU/mL".
- *Fetal abdominal measurements:* Measure proportion to the fetal head (head-to-abdominal circumference ratio: head bigger in 2nd trimester and early 3rd trimester).

- *Amniotic fluid index (AFI):* The sum of linear measurements (in centimeters) of the largest amniotic fluid pockets in each of the four quadrants. Normal values from 5 to 20 cm.
  - *AFI <5:* Oligohydramnios may be cord compression, fetal renal issues, associated with IUGR.
  - *AFI >20:* Polyhydramnios may be poorly controlled GDM or a fetal GI problem.
- *Amniotic fluid:* Protects from trauma and infection, aids in fetal lung development.
  - Normal volumes at 28 weeks—800 mL; at 40 weeks—500 mL.

ASSESSMENT OF FETAL WELLBEING

- Antepartum fetal surveillance may be conducted by a nonstress test (NST), fetal movement "kick counts," contraction stress test (CST), and the biophysical profile.
- Nonstress test is electronic fetal monitoring looking for reactivity to assess fetal wellbeing if fetal compromise is suspected.
  - *Reactive* is >2 accelerations in 20 minutes of ≥15 bpm above the baseline for at least 15 seconds. This is a healthy fetus.
  - *Nonreactive:* No accelerations detected in 40 minutes, follow with BPP (biophysical profile).
- *Kick counts:* Mom lies on her side and counts fetal movements. More than 10 movements within two hours is reassuring. Vibroacoustic stimulation or ingestion of food or caffeine can lightly stimulate the fetus to awaken it.

- A CST is done by infusing Oxytocin IV, to cause 3 contractions within 10 minutes.
  - Positive (nonreassuring) is late decelerations >50% of the contractions.
  - *Negative:* No late or significant variable decelerations.
  - *Equivocal:* Intermittent late or significant variable.
- Biophysical profile is an ultrasound evaluation of the fetus which awards two points each for fetal movement, fetal tone, fetal breathing, and an AFI >5 cm for a total of 8 points (10 points including a NST). A normal profile equals 8–10.

INTRAPARTUM FETAL MONITORING

- Interpret fetal heart rate (FHR) the same way every time for accuracy/consistency.
- First step is to determine the pregnancy risks
  - Low-risk, use intermittent or continuous monitoring of FHR and contractions.
  - In the first stage of labor, record or review strips every 30 minutes.
  - Second stage of labor, record or review strips every 15 minutes.
- In high-risk pregnancies, use only continuous electronic FHR and contraction monitoring.
  - With tracing review every 15 minutes during first stage.
  - And every 5 minutes during second stage.
  - Monitors can be internal (fetal scalp electrode) or external (transabdominal).

- *Baseline FHR:* Base rate over 10 minutes (not during contraction). Normal 110–160.
  - *Bradycardia:* It can be due to occipitoposterior position or postdates pregnancies.
  - *Tachycardia:* Maternal fever or dehydration, hyperthermia, fetal movement, anemia or immaturity.
  - Fetal tachycardia persistently over 180 + maternal fever may be chorioamnionitis.
- Variability refers to fluctuations in the baseline (not during contractions)
  - Absent—no detectable fluctuations: Maternal or fetal acidemia, asphyxia
  - Minimal—fluctuations less than 5 bpm
  - Moderate—fluctuations of 6–25 bpm (normal)
  - Marked—fluctuations over 25 bpm: Mild fetal hypoxemia.
- Look at the contraction number in 10 minutes. Normal <5.
- Tachysystole >5. For tachysystole, consider decreasing Oxytocin.
- Periodic FHR changes are accelerations/decelerations related to contractions.
- Accelerations are increases above baseline heart rate
  - Peaks within 30 seconds, and returns to baseline within 2 minutes.
  - Over 32 weeks gestation, heart rate gains >15 bpm and lasts for >15 seconds.
  - Under 32 weeks gestation, heart rate gains >10 bpm and lasts >10 seconds.

- If accelerations are not present, check fetal status with nonstress test, biophysical profile, or contractions stress test.
- Presence of accelerations correlates with a fetus that is not acidotic.
- Decelerations (decels) are the final element analyzed.
- Classification of fetal heart rate (FHR) tracings:
  - *Category I:* Normal tracing, normal FHR, moderate variability, no late or variable decels.
  - *Category II:* Intermediate, with tachycardia, any variability besides moderate, late or variable decels with moderate variability, prolonged decels, no accelerations.
    - *Management:* Check maternal vitals and cervix, maternal repositioning, give maternal oxygen and IV fluid bolus, stop Oxytocin, and consider amnioinfusion for suspected cord compression.
  - *Category III:* Consider immediate delivery. Sinusoidal pattern or absent variability with one of the following: recurrent late decels, recurrent variable decels or bradycardia.

DECELERATIONS IN DETAIL

Have different meaning depending on when they occur in relation to contractions.

- **Early decelerations** are normal and due to head compression with contractions.

- The timing of onset, peak and end of decel match those points in the contraction. The degree of deceleration is proportional to the contraction strength and is regulated by vagal nerve activation. No intervention is required.
- **Late decelerations** are abnormal and are due to uteroplacental insufficiency (not enough blood to the fetus during contractions). They begin at the peak of contraction and end slowly after the contraction has stopped. Intervention needed.
  - Change maternal position to lateral recumbent and give oxygen by face mask.
  - Stop Oxytocin (Pitocin) infusion and give an IV tocolytic drug ($MgSO_4$).
  - Monitor maternal blood pressure and give an IV fluid bolus.
  - If lasting >30 minutes, measure fetal scalp blood pH and consider C-section.
- **Variable decelerations** are abnormal and due to cord or head compression. Can be mild or severe and can occur at any time. If they are repetitive, suspect that the cord is wrapped around the neck or under the arm of the fetus. Intervention needed.
  - *Amnioinfusion:* Infuse normal saline into the uterus to alleviate cord compression.
  - Change maternal position to side/Trendelenburg position.
  - Deliver fetus with forceps or C-section.

- **Prolonged:** Lasts 2–10 minutes. Rule out cord prolapse and manage as late decelerations.

METABOLIC CHANGES IN PREGNANCY

- Body water increases by 8.5 L overall.
- Energy requirements increase during second trimester by 50–100 kcal/day. In third trimester, requirements are increased by 300 kcal/day.
- The uterus and placenta use carbohydrates, fats, and amino acids.
    - Insulin sensitivity rises and fasting glucose levels are lower in the first 20 weeks for fat and glycogen storage (anabolic state for building up reserves).
    - After 20 weeks, fasting glucose and insulin levels rise and insulin resistance develops (the fetus uses resistance to keep glucose for itself). Mom uses lipids for energy. Screen for gestational DM at 26–28 weeks.
- All lipid levels are elevated during pregnancy (lipids can cross the placenta).
    - As the mom has increased lipid use, lipoproteins have an increased rate of breakdown, leading to increased cholesterol (for energy and for steroid production).
    - Cholesterol levels can triple during pregnancy, and total cholesterol stays high even after delivery. Higher cholesterol levels increase overall risk of gallstones.
    - Triglycerides raise the most. Also higher are very low-density lipoprotein (VLDL), low-density lipoprotein (LDL), and high-density lipoprotein (HDL).

- LDL cholesterol is the main lipoprotein used in fetal adrenal steroidogenesis.
- Changes in body weight are maternal weight until the third trimester, when it is truly baby weight (fetal growth). Normal-weight moms should gain is 25–35 pounds total.

ENDOCRINE SYSTEM CHANGES

- In general, the endocrine system is modified by the placenta.
  - *Human chorionic gonadotropin (hCG):* Stimulates production of both adrenal and placental steroids. Causes fetal testes to secrete testosterone. Also stimulates thyroid growth.
  - *PL (human placental lactogen):* Anti-insulin and growth hormone-like effects → impaired maternal glucose utilization and free fatty acid release.
- *Thyroid gland:* Increases in size. Total thyroxine levels and thyroxine-binding globulin levels increase, so that the free thyroxine remains normal and the maternal free T4 levels do not actually change (mom stays euthyroid).
- *Parathyroid glands:* PTH increases to increase maternal calcium absorption. This provides replacement of the maternal calcium used by the fetus. Calcitonin is very high in the fetus for creation of fetal bone.
- Pancreas increases both in size and number of cells. Also the number of insulin receptor sites increases.
- *Glucagon:* Levels are slightly raised in pregnancy, but not as much as insulin levels.

- *Prolactin:* Levels raise beginning very early in pregnancy to up to 20 times higher than in nonpregnant women.
- *Adrenal gland:* Corticosteroids can reach 3–5 times nonpregnant levels due to increased production and decreased clearance.

STEROID CHANGES IN PREGNANCY

- Corticosteroid increase causes striae on the abdomen, breasts, etc.
- Estrogens affect uterine vasculature, the production of placental steroids, and the pregnancy.
  - Estradiol is produced by the maternal ovaries for the first 6 weeks of gestation. Then the production is in the placenta by converting circulating DHEA-S. After the first trimester, the placenta is the major source of circulating estradiol.
  - Estrone is produced in the maternal ovaries and adrenal glands, with peripheral conversion in the first 4–6 weeks of pregnancy. The placenta secretes increasing quantities after 6 weeks.
  - Estriol is produced in the placenta for as long as there is a living fetus present.
- Progesterone is produced by the corpus luteum before 6 weeks, and then the placenta takes over production from LDL cholesterol. The progesterone affects tubal motility, the endometrium, uterine vasculature, and inhibits T-lymphocyte–mediated tissue rejection.

- Decidual tissue makes cortisol which functions to decrease the maternal immune response to fetal tissue.

GASTROINTESTINAL SYSTEM CHANGES

- Gallbladder
  - Increases in size and empties more slowly. Also, there are increases in cholesterol which make patients more prone to gallstones.
  - Cholestasis occurs likely due to high estrogen and progesterone levels decreasing contractility.
- Liver
  - Liver function is increased. Albumin synthesis increases and the total albumin mass increases early in pregnancy, yet the concentration is overall decreased, causing peripheral edema.
  - Velocity of blood flow in hepatic veins decreases.
  - Serum alkaline phosphatase increases largely due to placental production.
- Reflux esophagitis (heartburn)
  - Enlarging uterus displaces the stomach above the esophageal sphincter and causes increased intra-gastric pressure.
  - Progesterone causes a relative relaxation of the esophageal sphincter.
  - There may also be reflux of bile into the stomach due to pyloric incompetence.
- Constipation may occur secondary to progesterone, which relaxes intestinal smooth muscle and slows peristalsis.

RESPIRATORY AND CARDIOVASCULAR CHANGES

- Respiratory changes:
  - Tidal volume and vital capacity increase.
  - Progesterone reduces the CO_2 threshold at which the respiratory center is stimulated. This causes increased breathing, known as hyperventilation of pregnancy.
- Cardiovascular changes:
  - Heart sounds:
    * At end of the first trimester, S1 becomes louder, with exaggerated splitting.
    * During second and third trimester, most women have a third heart sound or S3 gallop with the increases in volume.
    * Systolic ejection murmurs along the left sternal border occur in most patients (increased flow across aortic and pulmonic valves).
    * Diastolic murmurs are never normal—if detected, refer to cardiology.
  - Cardiac output increases by 60% overall (increased stroke volume and heart rate).
  - EKG changes from pre-pregnancy may not be ischemia. The heart dilates and the diaphragm rises, which changes its position relative to the electrodes.
  - Systemic vascular resistance steadily decreases.
    * In labor, central venous pressure increases by 3–5 mm Hg during each contraction.

Normal Pregnancy

❖ Diastolic blood pressure decreases during the second trimester, and increases during labor with the contractions. Systolic BP tends to stay the same.

HEMATOLOGIC CHANGES

- Plasma volume rises, increasing by 50% overall. RBC mass is only increased by 20-30%, so there is hemodilution. The reduced viscosity increases capillary blood flow, while the increased circulatory volume helps compensate for the increased blood flow to the uterus and kidneys.
- MCV begins to increase in the first trimester due to the expanding RBC mass.
  - *Erythrocyte sedimentation rate (ESR):* Rises early in pregnancy due to increased fibrinogen and other physiologic changes. An ESR of 100 mm/h is not uncommon.
- White blood cells:
  - Neutrophil count increases in T1 and continues to rise until 30 weeks. Neutrophilic metabolic activity and phagocytic function increases.
  - Lymphocyte counts remain unchanged, but their function is suppressed.
- Platelet reactivity is increased in T2 and T3 and returns to normal at 12 weeks postpartum. Platelet count may fall below 150,000 without effects on the fetus.

- Venous system:
  - Venous dilation results from relaxation of vascular smooth muscle as well as the pressure of enlarging uterus on inferior vena cava and iliac veins.
  - Predisposition to developing varicose veins of legs, vulva, rectum and pelvis.
  - The superior rectal vein is part of the portal system. As it does not have valves, the high system pressure produces hemorrhoids.

GENITOURINARY AND RENAL CHANGES

- Genitourinary (GU) system:
  - Urinary stasis occurs due to ureteral dilation from hormonal effects (mainly progesterone) and compression of the ureter at the pelvic brim as pregnancy progresses.
  - Urinating four times per night is normal; fetal movements, bladder compression and insomnia contribute to the nocturia.
  - Urinary frequency increases due to bladder compression. If the patient also has dysuria, hematuria, flank pain or suprapubic pain, evaluate for a UTI/cystitis or pyelonephritis.
  - Asymptomatic bacteriuria + urinary stasis predispose patients to pyelonephritis. Pregnancy is one of the few times that asymptomatic bacteriuria is treated.
  - Stress incontinence occurs due to relaxation of bladder supports. Bladder tone decreases due to the progesterone, but capacity increases.

- Renal system:
  - The ureters dilate up to the calyces and increase glomerular size. Urine flow rate decreases, while renal plasma flow increases. These changes lead to increased GFR and a fall in the serum creatinine. This means that a high normal serum creatinine may reflect renal impairment.
  - Tubules lose some of their absorption, so amino acids, uric acid and glucose are lost in the urine.
  - Plasma aldosterone increases and sodium retention causes peripheral edema.

CENTRAL NERVOUS SYSTEM AND SKIN CHANGES IN PREGNANCY

- Central nervous system (CNS):
  - *Syncope has many factors:* Venous pooling causes dizziness; dehydration; hypoglycemia; blood flow shunting to the stomach after eating; overexertion.
  - Emotional and psychiatric symptoms may result from hormonal changes of pregnancy. Progesterone can cause tiredness, dyspnea and depression. Endogenous corticosteroids can cause euphoria.
- Skin:
  - Melanocyte-stimulating hormone increases can cause—Linea nigra (dark line of the abdomen from above the umbilicus to the pubis); darkening of nipple and areola; facial melasma (hyperpigmentation in exposed areas such as the face).
  - Estrogen can cause—Spider nevi (branched growths of dilated capillaries on the skin) and palmar erythema.

BIBLIOGRAPHY

ACOG Committee on Practice Bulletins. ACOG Practice Bulletin No. 77: Screening for fetal chromosomal abnormalities. Obstet Gynecol 2007;109:217.

Almeida FA, Pavan MV, Rodrigues CI. The haemodynamic, renal excretory and hormonal changes induced by resting in the left lateral position in normal pregnant women during late gestation. BJOG 2009;116:1749.

American Academy of Pediatrics, American College of Obstetricians and Gynecologists. Guidelines for perinatal care (5th edn). Elk Grove Village, Ill.: AAP & ACOG; Washington, D.C, 2002.

American Academy of Pediatrics. Group B streptococcal infections. In: 2012 Report of the Committee on Infectious Diseases. Pickering LK. (Ed), American Academy of Pediatrics, Elk Grove Village, IL 2012; p.680.

American College of Obstetricians and Gynecologists Committee on Genetics. Committee Opinion No. 545: Noninvasive prenatal testing for fetal aneuploidy. Obstet Gynecol 2012;120:1532.

American College of Obstetricians and Gynecologists. ACOG Practice Bulletin No. 88, December 2007. Invasive prenatal testing for aneuploidy. Obstet Gynecol 2007;110:1459.

American College of Obstetricians and Gynecologists. ACOG Practice Bulletin No. 106: Intrapartum fetal heart rate monitoring: nomenclature, interpretation, and general management principles. Obstet Gynecol 2009;114:192.

American College of Obstetricians and Gynecologists. Practice bulletin No. 116: Management of intrapartum fetal heart rate tracings. Obstet Gynecol 2010;116:1232.

Normal Pregnancy

American Institute of Ultrasound in Medicine, Standards AIUM Practice Guideline for the performance of the antepartum obstetrical ultrasound examinations. American Institute of Ultrasound in Medicine, Laurel, MD 2007.

Artal R, Lockwood CJ, Brown HL. Weight gain recommendations in pregnancy and the obesity epidemic. Obstet Gynecol 2010;115:152.

Bailey R. Intrapartum Fetal Monitoring. Am Fam Physicia. 2009:15;[80(12)]:1388-96.

Battagliarin G, Lanna M, Coviello D, et al. A randomized study to assess two different techniques of aspiration while performing transabdominal chorionic villus sampling. Ultrasound Obstet Gynecol 2009;33:169.

Berghella V, Baxter JK, Chauhan SP. Evidence-based labor and delivery management. Am J Obstet Gynecol 2008;199:445.

Bernstein IM, Ziegler W, Badger GJ. Plasma volume expansion in early pregnancy. Obstet Gynecol 2001;97:669.

Berry SM, Stone J, et al. Society for Maternal-Fetal Medicine (SMFM). Fetal blood sampling. Am J Obstet Gynecol 2013;209:170.

Biedenbach DJ, Stephen JM, Jones RN. Antimicrobial susceptibility profile among beta-haemolytic Streptococcus spp. collected in the SENTRY Antimicrobial Surveillance Program—North America, 2001. Diagn Microbiol Infect Dis. 2003;46:291.

Bradley CS, Kennedy CM, Turcea AM, et al. Constipation in pregnancy: prevalence, symptoms, and risk factors. Obstet Gynecol 2007;110:1351.

Canick JA, Lambert-Messerlian GM, Palomaki GE, et al. Comparison of serum markers in first-trimester down syndrome screening. Obstet Gynecol 2006;108:1192.

Centers for Disease Control and Prevention (CDC). Perinatal group B streptococcal disease after universal screening recommendations—United States, 2003-2005. MMWR Morb Mortal Wkly Rep 2007;56:701.

Clapp JF 3rd, Seaward BL, Sleamaker RH, Hiser J. Maternal physiologic adaptations to early human pregnancy. Am J Obstet Gynecol 1988;159:1456.

Clark SL, Cotton DB, Lee W, et al. Central hemodynamic assessment of normal term pregnancy. Am J Obstet Gynecol 1989;161:1439.

Del Valle GO, Joffe GM, Izquierdo LA, et al. The biophysical profile and the nonstress test: poor predictors of chorioamnionitis and fetal infection in prolonged preterm premature rupture of membranes. Obstet Gynecol 1992;80:106.

Depp, R. Cesarean delivery. In: Gabbe, SG, Niebyl, JR, Simpson, JL (Eds). Obstetrics. Normal and Problem Pregnancies, 4th edn, Churchill Livingstone: New York, 2002, p. 551.

Dörr HG, Heller A, Versmold HT, et al. Longitudinal study of progestins, mineralocorticoids, and glucocorticoids throughout human pregnancy. J Clin Endocrinol Metab. 1989;68:863.

Geraghty LN, Pomeranz MK. Physiologic changes and dermatoses of pregnancy. Int J Dermatol 2011;50:771.

Glinoer D. What happens to the normal thyroid during pregnancy? Thyroid 1999;9:631.

Graves, CR. Acute pulmonary complications in pregnancy. In: Fink, MP, Abraham, E, Vincent, J, Kochanek, PM (Eds), Textbook of Critical Care, Elsevier Saunders: Philadelphia, 2005. p.1551.

Grindheim G, Estensen ME, Langesaeter E, et al. Changes in blood pressure during healthy pregnancy: a longitudinal cohort study. J Hypertens 2012;30:342.

Heenan AP, Wolfe LA, Davies GA, McGrath MJ. Effects of human pregnancy on fluid regulation responses to short-term exercise. J Appl Physiol 2003;95:2321.

Herrera E. Metabolic adaptations in pregnancy and their implications for the availability of substrates to the fetus. Eur J Clin Nutr 2000;54 (Suppl 1):S47.

Hill LM, Guzick D, Hixson J, et al. Composite assessment of gestational age: a comparison of institutionally derived and published regression equations. Am J Obstet Gynecol 1992;166:551.

Jackson AA. Nutrients, growth, and the development of programmed metabolic function. Adv Exp Med Biol 2000;478:41.

Klajnbard A, Szecsi PB, Colov NP, et al. Laboratory reference intervals during pregnancy, delivery and the early postpartum period. Clin Chem Lab Med 2010;48:237.

Kupesic Plavsic S, et al. Normal Pregnancy. Video Atlas of Clinical Skills in Ob Gyn, New Delhi: Jaypee Publisher, 2012.

Lanham M, Morgan H. University of Michigan OB-Gyn Survival Guide, 2011.

Larsson A, Palm M, Hansson LO, Axelsson O. Reference values for clinical chemistry tests during normal pregnancy. BJOG 2008;115:874.

Lewis DF, Adair CD, Weeks JW, et al. A randomized clinical trial of daily nonstress testing versus biophysical profile in the management of preterm premature rupture of membranes. Am J Obstet Gynecol 1999;181:1495.

Macones GA, Hankins GD, Spong CY, Hauth J, Moore T. The 2008 National Institute of Child Health and Human Development workshop report on electronic fetal monitoring: update on definitions, interpretation, and research guidelines. Obstet Gynecol 2008;112(3):661-6.

Maldonado D, Zuniga C, Uzelac P. SOAP for Family Medicine. Lippincott Williams & Wilkins, 2005.pp.70-1.

Manning FA, Morrison I, Lange IR, et al. Fetal biophysical profile scoring: selective use of the nonstress test. Am J Obstet Gynecol 1987;156:709.

Mastorakos G, Ilias I. Maternal hypothalamic-pituitary-adrenal axis in pregnancy and the postpartum period. Postpartum-related disorders. Ann N Y Acad Sci 2000;900:95.

Matthews SG, Gibb W, Lye SJ. Endocrine and paracrine regulation of birth at term and preterm. Endocr Rev 2000;21:514.

McAuliffe F, Kametas N, Costello J, et al. Respiratory function in singleton and twin pregnancy. BJOG 2002;109:765.

McIntyre HD, Chang AM, Callaway LK, et al. Hormonal and metabolic factors associated with variations in insulin sensitivity in human pregnancy. Diabetes Care 2010;33:356.

Mintz MC, Grumbach K, Arger PH, Coleman BG. Sonographic evaluation of bile duct size during pregnancy. AJR Am J Roentgenol 1985;145:575.

Moise KJ Jr, Argoti PS. Management and prevention of red cell alloimmunization in pregnancy: a systematic review. Obstet Gynecol 2012;120:1132.

Nel JT, Diedericks A, Joubert G, Arndt K. A prospective clinical and urodynamic study of bladder function during and after pregnancy. Int Urogynecol J Pelvic Floor Dysfunct 2001;12:21.

Nevo O, Soustiel JF, Thaler I. Maternal cerebral blood flow during normal pregnancy: a cross-sectional study. Am J Obstet Gynecol 2010;203:475.e1.

Norwitz E, Robinson J, Repke J. Labor and delivery. In: Gabbe SG, Niebyl JR, Simpson JL (Eds). Obstetrics: normal and problem pregnancies, 4th edn. New York: Churchill Livingstone; 2002. pp.353-94.

Parer JT, Ikeda T. A framework for standardized management of intrapartum fetal heart rate patterns. Am J Obstet Gynecol 2007;197:26.e1.

Prasad MR, Krugh D, Rossi KQ, O'Shaughnessy RW. Anti-D in Rh positive pregnancies. Am J Obstet Gynecol 2006;195:1158.

Preventing group B streptococcal infections: New recommendations. Paediatr Child Health 2002;6:380-3.

Reddy UM, Mennuti MT. Incorporating first-trimester Down syndrome studies into prenatal screening: executive summary of the National

Institute of Child Health and Human Development workshop. Obstet Gynecol 2006;107:167.

Reis FM, D'Antona D, Petraglia F. Predictive value of hormone measurements in maternal and fetal complications of pregnancy. Endocr Rev 2002;23:230.

Rey E, Rodriguez-Artalejo F, Herraiz MA, et al. Gastroesophageal reflux symptoms during and after pregnancy: a longitudinal study. Am J Gastroenterol 2007;102:2395.

Sandler SG, Li W, Langeberg A, Landy HJ. New laboratory procedures and Rh blood type changes in a pregnant woman. Obstet Gynecol 2012;119:426.

Schrag S, Gorwitz R, Fultz-Butts K, Schuchat A. Prevention of perinatal group B streptococcal disease. Revised guidelines from CDC. MMWR Recomm Rep 2002;51:1.

Sekulić SR. Possible explanation of cephalic and noncephalic presentation during pregnancy: a theoretical approach. Med Hypotheses 2000;55:429.

U.S. Department of Health and Human Services, Office on Women's Health. Prenatal Care Fact Sheet, March, 2009.

University Hospitals Case Medical Center, MacDonald Women's Hospital. Resident's Manual, 2007.

van Brummen HJ, Bruinse HW, van der Bom JG, et al. How do the prevalences of urogenital symptoms change during pregnancy? Neurourol Urodyn 2006;25:135.

Vaughan Jones SA, Black MM. Pregnancy dermatoses. J Am Acad Dermatol 1999;40:233.

Verani JR, McGee L, Schrag SJ. Prevention of perinatal group B streptococcal disease—revised guidelines from CDC 2010. MMWR Recomm Rep 2010;59:1.

Wesnes SL, Rortveit G, Bø K, Hunskaar S. Urinary incontinence during pregnancy. Obstet Gynecol 2007;109:922.

Westerway SC, Davison A, Cowell S. Ultrasonic fetal measurements: new Australian standards for the new millennium. Aust N Z J Obstet Gynaecol 2000;40(3):297-302.

Westgate JA, Wibbens B, Bennet L, et al. The intrapartum deceleration in center stage: a physiologic approach to the interpretation of fetal heart rate changes in labor. Am J Obstet Gynecol 2007;197:236.e1.

Wijma J, Potters AE, de Wolf BT, et al. Anatomical and functional changes in the lower urinary tract following spontaneous vaginal delivery. BJOG 2003;110:658.

World Health Organization, Maternal and Newborn Health/Safe Motherhood Unit. Care in Normal Birth: A Practical Guide, 1996; http://www.who.int/maternal_child_adolescent/documents/who_frh_msm_9624/en

Youssef A, Ghi T, Pilu G. How to perform ultrasound in labor: assessment of fetal occiput position. Ultrasound Obstet Gynecol 2013;41:476.

2
Pregnancy Complications

CHAPTER OUTLINES

- Triage Tips
- Sample Triage/Labor and Delivery H+P Note
- Gestational Diabetes Mellitus
- HIV in Pregnancy
- Intrauterine Growth Restriction
- Thyroid in Pregnancy
- Epilepsy
- Abdominal and Renal Disorders
- Gestational Hypertension
- Pre-eclampsia
- Eclampsia
- Antihypertensive/Anticonvulsant Doses
- Hemolysis, Elevated Liver Enzymes, Low Platelets Syndrome
- Thrombosis
- Peripartum Cardiomyopathy
- First Trimester Bleeding
- Third Trimester Bleeding
- Ectopic Pregnancy
- Placenta Previa
- Placental Abruption
- Uterine Rupture
- Vasa Previa
- Fetal Demise
- Induced Abortion
- Abortion Methods
- Medications in Pregnancy
- Antibiotics, Androgens and Pain Medications
- Asthmatic and Cardiovascular Medications

TRIAGE TIPS

- For all patients assess for FM, VB, LOF, and contractions. Review prenatal records and dating. All triage patients should have electronic fetal monitoring.

- *In case of decreased fetal movement:* Estimate fetal weight, and check NST. If not reactive, get BPP.
- Ask about abdominal pain, dysuria, and gastric problems. Remember pregnant women can have appendicitis, gallbladder disorders, GERD, etc.
- *Round ligament pain:* Considered normal. Occurs at about 20–30 weeks and radiates to the groin. Shifting the uterus from the left to the right can reproduce it.
- *Low back pain:* Determine if it is related to contractions, musculoskeletal or CVA tenderness.
- *Nausea and vomiting:* Consider hyperemesis gravidarum, viral gastroenteritis, UTI/pyelonephritis. Is patient dehydrated?
- *Swelling:* Edema can be normal, but swelling in the face or rapid weight gain associated with water retention could be a sign of pre-eclampsia. Evaluate blood pressure and consider pre-eclampsia work-up.
- *Recognize signs of labor:* Look for regular contractions with cervical change. If preterm, consider fetal fibronectin (fFN) prior to cervical exam. If no ROM or bleeding, serial vaginal exams assessing for cervical changes. Consider UTI, dehydration, etc.
- *Rupture of membranes (ROM):* Perform speculum exam looking for pooling of fluid, loss of fluid from cervix with Valsalva, place fluid on slide to look for ferning (arborization). Place fluid on nitrazine strip for nitrazine test. If tests are equivocal or negative but strong clinical suspicion remains, order US for AFI.
- *Vaginal bleeding:* Do not perform SVE without knowing location of placenta. Perform sterile speculum exam or transabdominal ultrasound. Bleeding can also be related to

extropion or eversion of the endocervix, which is more friable and can bleed, particularly after intercourse.

SAMPLE TRIAGE/LABOR AND DELIVERY H+P NOTE

- *Chief complaint (CC):* Leakage of fluid, contractions, vaginal bleeding, abdominal pain, etc.
- *History of present illness (HPI):* __ yo G__P__ @ __-__/7 weeks by LMP (consistent with 1st trimester US) presents with ____ +/- FM, LOF, VB, contractions, HA, vision changes, RUQ pain.
- Pregnancy complicated by _____. Prenatal care @ _____.
- *LMP:* _____ EDD: _____
- *OB Hx:* G_P_ (year; term or preterm, if preterm-why; vaginal or cesarean, type of cesarean and why; male of female; weight; complications, GA of abortions).
- *GYN Hx:* h/o STDs, abnormal Paps, etc.
- *Past medical history (PMH):* ____ PSH: ____ Meds: PNV Allergies: ___ (always NOTE reaction).
- *Family Hx:* Include birth defects as well as bleeding or clotting disorders.
- *Social Hx:* +/- tobacco, EtOH, drugs. Living situation, occupation, Hx of depression.
- *Review of systems (ROS):* _____
- *Physical examination (PE):* Mother's vitals, baby's vitals: analysis of fetal monitoring strips, contractions pattern and frequency.
- *Sterile speculum exam (SSE):* Bleeding or pooling, cervix visually dilated to ___ cm
- *Sterile vaginal exam (SVE):* Dilation/%, effacement, station.

GESTATIONAL DIABETES MELLITUS

- Pregestational diabetes—patient had DM before pregnancy.
- Gestational diabetes—patient develops diabetes only during pregnancy.
- Glucose challenge screening test—done at 26–28 weeks. Human placental lactogen plays a pivotal role in triggering the changes that can lead to glucose intolerance in pregnancy.
    - Give 50 mg glucose (nonfasting). Draw glucose blood level 1 hour later.
    - If ≥200, patient is diagnosed with gestational diabetes mellitus (GDM) type A1 and a diabetic diet is started.
    - If >140 but <200 then perform a 3-hour glucose tolerance test:
        * Draw fasting glucose level; (normal (n) <95), then give 100 g glucose load.
        * Draw glucose levels at 1 hour (n <180), 2 hours (n < 155), and at 3 hours (n <140).
        * Positive for gestational diabetes if 2/4 values are high.

GDM increases risk of maternal pre-eclampsia, maternal bacterial infections, C-section, polyhydramnios, birth injury, perinatal death, fetal anomalies (renal, cardiac, and CNS), preterm delivery, fetal macrosomia, birth injury and fetal metabolic derangements (hypoglycemia, hypocalcemia).

- *GDMA1:* Diet controlled
- *GDMA2:* Medication controlled
- *Management:*
    - Maintain good glucose control with either insulin or diet. Keep fasting sugars <95 and 2 hours postprandial sugars <120. If >50% of sugars higher than this range, change therapy at check-up.

- Perform ultrasonography to rule out fetal macrosomia and evaluate fetal growth, estimated weight, amniotic fluid volume, and fetal anatomy at 16 to 20 weeks' GA.
  - *Starting at 32 to 34 weeks:* Nonstress test and amniotic fluid index testing weekly to biweekly depending on disease severity.
  - If fetal weight is >4,500 g, consider elective C-section to avoid shoulder dystocia.
  - Check a 75 g two hours GTT at 6–8 weeks postpartum to monitor the patients for diabetes.

HIV IN PREGNANCY

- Majority of neonatal AIDS are secondary to transmission from mother to fetus.
- At the preconception visit, encourage maternal HIV screening.
- Reduced maternal viral load will reduce intrapartum transmission. Start antiretroviral therapy (ART) beginning after 12 weeks.
- Monitor CD4+ counts every 3 months and viral loads monthly till viral RNA is undetectable.
- Monitor monthly blood counts and liver functions while on ART.
- HIV RNA should be assessed at 34–36 weeks GA to determine the mode of delivery.
- Reduce peripartum exposure by reducing duration of ruptured membranes.
- Intravenous (IV) Zidovudine should be administered to HIV-infected women with HIV RNA ≥400 copies/mL (or unknown HIV RNA) near delivery, regardless of antepartum regimen or mode of delivery.

- IV Zidovudine is not required for HIV-infected women receiving combination antiretroviral (ARV) regimens who have HIV RNA <400 copies/mL near delivery.
- Scheduled cesarean delivery at 38 weeks' gestation is recommended for women with HIV RNA levels >1,000 copies/mL or unknown HIV levels near the time of delivery, irrespective of administration of antepartum ARV drugs.
- Scheduled cesarean delivery is not recommended for prevention of perinatal transmission in pregnant women receiving combination ARV drugs with plasma HIV RNA levels <1,000 copies/mL near time of delivery.
- Administer newborn prophylaxis for 6 weeks.

INTRAUTERINE GROWTH RESTRICTION

- Defined as growth at <10% tile. Significant morbidity and mortality are noticed at growth restriction <3% tile.
- Causes:
    - Decreased oxygen or nutrition from the placenta
    - High altitudes, multiple gestation, placental defects, pre-eclampsia/eclampsia
    - Congenital or chromosomal abnormalities and fetal infections (TORCH)
    - *Maternal risks:* Alcohol or drug abuse, clotting disorders, hypertension, kidney disease, poor nutrition, and smoking.
- Types
    - *Asymmetric:* Most common form. Due to a restriction of weight, then length, while the head circumference grows at normal rates. Typically occurs with problems in the third trimester, commonly pre-eclampsia.

- *Symmetric:* Less common and more worrisome. The whole fetus is generally small and signifies that the fetus has developed slowly through the whole pregnancy. These fetuses are more likely to have permanent neurologic sequelae. Common causes are infections, chromosomal abnormalities and anemia.
- Management includes modified bed rest, growth US every 3–4 weeks, fetal artery Doppler measurements (GA <35 weeks), twice weekly antenatal testing, and steroids and early delivery when indicated.
- *Note:* Small for gestational age (SGA) can only be diagnosed after delivery.

THYROID IN PREGNANCY

- *Hyperthyroid:* Graves' is the most common cause of thyrotoxicosis in pregnancy.
    - *Treatment is with medication:* Propylthiouracil/Methimazole or surgery. Radioactive iodine is contraindicated in pregnancy.
    - Thyroid storm is a major risk. Precipitating factors include infection, labor, and C-section. Treat with: beta-blocker, sodium iodide, parathyroid hormone (PTH) and dexamethasone.
    - Carries a 1% risk of neonatal thyrotoxicosis. Possible complications are: fetal goiter/hypothyroid, usually from PTU, preterm delivery and pre-eclampsia.
- Hypothyroidism
    - Subclinical hypothyroidism (elevated TSH but normal T4) is more common than overt hypothyroidism (elevated TSH and low T4), and often goes unnoticed.

- Postpartum thyroiditis
    - Transient postpartum hypothyroidism or thyrotoxicosis associated with autoimmune thyroiditis is common.
    - From 1–4 months postpartum, 4% of all women develop transient thyrotoxicosis.
    - Between 4 and 8 months postpartum, 2 to 5% of all women develop hypothyroidism.
- Sheehan syndrome
    - Pituitary ischemia and necrosis associated with obstetrical blood loss leading to hypopituitarism. Patients do not lactate postpartum due to low PRL.

EPILEPSY

- Epileptic women taking anticonvulsants during pregnancy have double the risk of malformations and pre-eclampsia. Women with a convulsive disorder that do not take medications still have an increased risk of birth defects.
    - Pregnant epileptics are more prone to seizures due to the associated stress and fatigue of pregnancy.
    - The fetus is at risk for megaloblastic anemia.
    - The pregnant female and her fetus are at risk for hemorrhage due to a deficiency of vitamin K-dependent clotting factors induced by anticonvulsant drugs.
- Management of the epileptic female should begin with pre pregnancy counseling. Once pregnant, the patient should be screened for neural tube defects and congenital malformations.
    - Anticonvulsant therapy should be reduced to the minimum effective dose of the minimum number of anticonvulsant medications.

- Women on anticonvulsants should be started on folic acid supplementation (5 mg/day).
- Blood levels of anticonvulsant medications should be checked at the beginning of pregnancy to determine the drug level that controls epileptic episodes successfully.

ABDOMINAL AND RENAL DISORDERS

- *Acute pyelonephritis:* Most common serious medical complication of pregnancy. Pregnancy causes hydronephrosis (dilatation of renal pelvis, calyces, and ureters) from compression and hormonal decreases in ureteral tone. This leads to urinary stasis and increased vesicoureteral reflux.
    - *Management:* Hospitalization, IV antibiotics (Ampicillin or Cefazolin) and monitor fluids status.
- *Acute abdomen in pregnancy*
    - During advanced pregnancy, GI symptoms become difficult to assess and the enlarged uterus often obscures physical findings.
- *Appendicitis* is the most common surgical condition in pregnancy.
    - Have usual symptoms, however, the uterus displaces the appendix superiorly and laterally. Pain and tenderness may not be found at McBurney's point (RLQ).
    - Rupture is more frequent in the third trimester as it is harder to recognize.
    - Management is appendectomy.
- *Cholecystitis*
    - Medical management unless common bile duct obstruction or pancreatitis develops, if this happens, cholecystectomy should be performed.

- Patient with cholecystitis have high risk of preterm labor.

GESTATIONAL HYPERTENSION

- Hypertension during pregnancy (in patients who were normotensive before 20 weeks):
    - *Mild:* Systolic BP ≥140 mm Hg and/or diastolic ≥ 90 mm Hg
    - *Severe:* Systolic BP >160 mm Hg and/or diastolic >110 mm Hg
- Subsets of gestational hypertension:
    - Simple gestational hypertension
    - *Pre-eclampsia:* Renal involvement leads to proteinuria.
    - *Eclampsia:* Central nervous system involvement leads to seizures.
    - *HELLP syndrome:* Dominated by hematologic and hepatic manifestations.
- *Complications:* Heart failure; cerebral hemorrhage; placental abruption; fetal growth restriction; fetal death
- Management:
    - *Mild:* Observe, bed rest
    - *Severe:* Always hospitalize + antihypertensive pharmacotherapy (Hydralazine or Labetalol for short-term control, Nifedipine or Methyldopa for long-term control).
    - Avoid ACE-I, ARBs, Atenolol and Thiazide diuretics – cause IUGR, oligohydramnios, neonatal renal failure and fetal death.
- The only cure of hypertensive disorders in pregnancy is delivery:
    - If >36 weeks and fetal lung mature: Induce labor.

- *If < 34 weeks/fetal lungs immature:* Steroids plus expectant management.
- If fetal or maternal deterioration or end organ signs at any gestational age, induce labor.

PRE-ECLAMPSIA

- Gestational hypertension with proteinuria. Rarely develops before 20 weeks.
- Subsets of pre-eclampsia:
  - *Mild:* BP: ≥140/90 with proteinuria: 300 mg to 5 g/24 hours
  - *Severe:* BP >160/110, proteinuria: >5 g/24 hours, high serum Cr, Oliguria (<500 mL/day). If end organ signs present, is automatically severe category.
- *End organ signs:* Headache, visual disturbances, epigastric/right upper quadrant pain, pulmonary edema, hepatocellular dysfunction (elevated AST and ALT), thrombocytopenia, IUGR, oligohydramnios, microangiopathic hemolysis, grand mal seizures (eclampsia).
- *Risk factors:* Nulliparity, history of pre-eclampsia or eclampsia, multiple fetuses, diabetes, vascular disease, renal disease, hydatidiform mole, fetal hydrops.
- Work-up:
  - *Blood:* Electrolytes, blood urea nitrogen (BUN), creatinine, liver function tests (LFTs) (ALT, AST), complete blood count (CBC), uric acid, and platelet count.
  - *Urine:* Sediment, 24 hours protein + creatinine, fetal US, non-stress test (NST), biophysical profile.
- Management:
  - *Mild:* Biweekly BP checks, lab and urinalysis, US to follow fetal growth, NST. Low-salt diet, monitor labs closely and deliver after 37 weeks.

- *Severe pre-eclampsia:* Hospitalize, bed rest, low salt, and low calories.
- *BP control:* Hydralazine or Labetalol short-term, Nifedipine or Methyldopa long-term.
- *Anticonvulsive therapy:* Magnesium sulfate.

ECLAMPSIA

- *Loss of regulation of cerebral blood flow:* Life-threatening. Aim is to prevent maternal injury.
- Do not use Diazepam or Phenytoin as they can cause respiratory depression/arrest, aspiration, and would not prevent recurrent eclamptic seizures.
  - *Control of the convulsions:* Mg sulfate 4–6 g load in 100 mL fluid, followed by 2 g/hr slowly.
  - Correction of hypoxia and acidosis
  - BP control (Hydralazine or Labetalol)
  - Delivery after control of convulsions
- Most eclampsia-related mortality is due to prematurity, growth restriction and placental abruption. In a seizure the fetus may have hypoxia-related bradycardia.

ANTIHYPERTENSIVE/ANTICONVULSANT DOSES

- If systolic blood pressure >160, or diastolic blood pressure >110:
  - Give IV Hydralazine 5 to 10 mg IV every 15–30 min (goal <160/100).
  - Or Labetalol 20 mg IV, if over goal in 10 min give 40 mg, over goal in 10 min give 80 mg max 220 mg in 1 hour (300 max/24 h).

- *Magnesium sulfate:* Loading dose 4-6 g given over 15-20 min followed by 2 g/h.
  - ❖ Check Mg levels 4 hours after load (goal 4-7 mg/dL)
  - ❖ Monitor reflexes, mental and respiratory status and urine output.
  - ❖ Keep 1g calcium gluconate at bedside in case of respiratory depression.

HEMOLYSIS, ELEVATED LIVER ENZYMES, LOW PLATELETS SYNDROME

- *Hemolysis:* Serum bilirubin >1.2, LDH >600, blood smear showing damaged RBCs.
- *Elevated LFTs:* AST >70, ALT >40, LDH >600.
- *Low platelets:* <100,000 (class 1 <50, class 2 50-100,000, class 3 100-150,000).
- HELLP syndrome is associated with:
  - High morbidity, multiparous mothers, mothers >25 years old, <36 weeks gestation.
- Presents as RUQ or epigastric pain, nausea and vomiting. Some have headache and visual changes. Coagulopathy can cause hematuria or GI bleeding.
  - Any patient who complains of RUQ/epigastric pain, N/V or signs of pre-eclampsia should be evaluated with CBC, platelet count and measurement of liver enzymes.
  - If platelets <50,000 or with active bleeding, measure fibrinogen, fibrin split products or d-dimer, PT/PTT to rule out superimposed DIC.
- Management
  - Treat pre-eclampsia, continue Mg until 24-48 hours after delivery.

- Corticosteroids only for lung maturity in pregnancies <34 weeks.
- Deliver infants >28 weeks gestation 24–48 hours after dexamethasone.
- FFP, platelets and PRBCs to correct coagulation deficits or hemorrhage.
- If patient develops shock and massive ascites, rule out spontaneous rupture of a subcapsular liver hematoma. Confirm with CT or US, and if positive, treat with emergent laparotomy.
- *Acute fatty liver of pregnancy:* Mildly low platelets and fatty liver (rare).
  - Deliver baby.

THROMBOSIS

- Risk of venous thromboembolism in pregnancy is 5 times nonpregnant risk.
  - Leading cause of maternal mortality in the US.
  - Includes both deep vein thrombosis (DVT) and pulmonary embolus (PE).
- Normal risk factors for thrombosis are present in every pregnancy
  - *Hypercoagulability:* Increased factor II, VII, X and fibrin, decreased protein S
  - *Stasis:* Pregnant uterus causes obstruction of inferior vena cava and venous distention
  - Vascular damage occurs with delivery
- *Deep vein thrombosis:* Unilateral leg pain and swelling. Order Doppler US of lower extremities.

- If thrombosis is detected, give therapeutic anticoagulation with LMWH.
- *Pulmonary embolism:* 2/3 occur in postpartum; presents as dyspnea, tachypnea, hypoxia.
  - Spiral CT scan or VQ scan (d-dimer is only useful if V/Q is negative).
  - Stabilize airway, breathing and circulation. Start anticoagulation as soon as suspected.
  - LMWH (Enoxaparin and Dalteparin), UFH (unfractionated Heparin) used while unstable.
- *Therapeutic anticoagulation in pregnancy:* Do not use warfarin (crosses placenta)
  - *LMWH:* Lovenox 1 mg/kg subcutaneous every 12 hours. As effective as Heparin, less side effects (thrombocytopenia, osteoporosis, bleeding, allergy); follow platelet counts
  - Heparin 5000 IU IV bolus, then 1300 IU/h IV or 15–20000 IU subcutaneous every 12 hours, INR every 6 hours × 4 then daily until therapeutic then weekly.
- *Prophylaxis:* 40 mg Lovenox sq daily (if >90 kg, twice daily). Heparin 5000 IU sq BID in first trimester, 7500 IU BID second trimester, 10000 IU sq BID third trimester.

PERIPARTUM CARDIOMYOPATHY

- Heart failure within 5 months of delivery or in the last month of pregnancy without any other identifiable cause.
  - Cause is unknown—genetics, inflammatory or autoimmune have been suggested
- Echo will show left ventricular systolic dysfunction.

- Symptoms of systolic dysfunction are dyspnea, fatigue, tachypnea and lower extremity edema. All are common in normal late pregnancy and so may not be recognized in a timely manner.
- 5th leading cause of maternal mortality in the US.
- *Risk factors include:* African descent, history of gestational hypertension, and multiparity
- Risk increases with age.
  - Management is not standard CHF therapy, as ACE-inhibitors should not be used in pregnancy, and diuretics can lead to ureteroplacental insufficiency.
  - Should be managed by cardiologists, with beta blockers or Digoxin
  - Prognosis depends on the degree of myocardial dysfunction
  - If cardiac function does not fully recover, women should avoid becoming pregnant again.

FIRST TRIMESTER BLEEDING

- *Evaluation:* Vital signs (rule out shock/sepsis/illness), Pelvic exam (look at cervix, source of bleed), β-hCG level, CBC, antibody screen, US (assess fetal viability).
- Spontaneous abortion is any type of loss of pregnancy before 20 weeks
  - *Causes:* Chromosomal abnormalities, infection, uterine abnormalities and/or anomalies, endocrine problems (PCOS/diabetes), immunologic factors (lupus anticoagulant/anticardiolipin), smoking or alcohol

- Stabilize patient with intravenous fluids (IVF). Give Oxytocin if heavy bleeding in present. Type and crossmatch for transfusion; give RhoGAM if mom is Rh negative; karyotype in patients with recurrent pregnancy loss.
- Evaluate for coagulopathy (fibrinogen, PTT, antibody screen).
- *Types of spontaneous abortion:*
    - *Incomplete:* Heavy bleeding and cramping with a dilated internal os but not all products have passed. Perform D&C.
    - *Septic:* Maternal infections cause fetal demise. Perform blood and cervical cultures, and D&C.
    - *Complete:* Heavy bleeding with tissue flow and no products of conception left in the uterus. If 8–14 weeks perform D&C as likely incomplete passage of products.
    - *Inevitable:* Bleeding with dilated cervix but no tissue has passed, often with cramping pain. Perform D&C.
    - *Missed abortion:* Fetus/embryo without heart tones but no tissue is passed and internal cervical os closed. Perform D&C or Oxytocin with cervical dilation.
    - *Threatened abortion:* Vaginal bleeding in the first 20 weeks, internal cervical os not open and no rupture of membranes. Observation, bed rest and pelvic rest. 50% result in pregnancy loss.

THIRD TRIMESTER BLEEDING

- Evaluation
    - History and physical; vitals; labs: CBC, coagulation profile, type and cross, urinalysis

- Determine whether blood is maternal or fetal or both:
  - *Apt test:* Put blood from vagina in tube with KOH: brown is maternal, pink is fetal.
  - *Kleihauer–Betke test:* Take blood from mother's arm and determine percentage of fetal RBCs in maternal circulation: >1% indicates fetal bleeding.
  - *Wright's stain:* Vaginal blood; nucleated RBCs indicate fetal bleed.
- Causes of late pregnancy bleeding
  - *Life-threatening:* Placenta previa, placental abruption, vasa previa and uterine rupture.
  - *Less serious:* Cervicitis, cervical polyps, cervical neoplasm, and bloody show.
- Management
  - If there is heavy bleeding, stabilize the mother, acquire baseline labs. If the mother has DIC or if unable to stabilize the mom, deliver the baby.
  - If she does not have DIC, once mom is stabilized, is the fetal strip reassuring?
- If not, reposition the mom, check blood pressure, IV and tocolysis
- If the fetal strip still not reassuring, possible vasa previa, deliver the baby.
- If the fetal strip normalizes, evaluate the positioning of the placenta. Low placenta may be placenta previa. If placenta is not low, rule out placental abruption. Manage conservatively and observe.

ECTOPIC PREGNANCY

- Implantation anywhere other than inside the uterine cavity. EP is a medical emergency, caused by malfunction in fallopian tube transport due to:
  - Infection (*Chlamydia* and gonorrhea); abdominal surgery (adhesions); endometriosis, and other causes
  - Consider other locations of ectopic pregnancy such as cervical, cornual, abdominal and ovarian
- *Signs:* Adnexal tenderness or mass; lack of intrauterine gestation on US; subnormal values of hCG and/or plateau; low serum progesterone level (<25 ng/mL).
- *Transvaginal ultrasound is diagnostic if:* Gestational sac is seen outside of uterus, if any adnexal mass (excluding corpus luteum) is seen, or if pelvic free fluid seen. Ectopic ruled out if intrauterine pregnancy is seen (very rare-heterotopic pregnancy has one intrauterine and one extrauterine pregnancy).
  - If US not definitive, measure serum hCG. If above 1,500, should be able to visualize an intrauterine gestational sac. Recheck serum hCG in 48 hours to assess hCG trend (in normal intrauterine pregnancy hCG doubles every 48 hours).
- Manage
  - *Expectant:* If hCG <1,000 and falling, minimal pain or adnexal mass <3 cm.
  - *Medical:* If hCG <5,000 and patient is stable, give 1 mg/kg IM Methotrexate and recheck hCG every 7 days.

- Operative if unstable vital signs, uncertain diagnosis, advanced ectopic pregnancy, unsure of follow-up, any contraindication to methotrexate, or hCG not falling with MTX.
- If ectopic pregnancy ruptures, it usually presents as shock. Stabilize with IV fluids, blood transfusion, and pressors if necessary. Operative treatment is necessary with rupture of ectopic pregnancy.

PLACENTA PREVIA

- Placenta is implanted close to the cervix. Presents as painless, profuse bleeding in the second and/or third trimester, or earlier with spotting, postcoital bleeding or cramping. Three types of placenta previa:
  1. *Complete placenta previa:* The placenta covers the entire internal cervical os.
  2. *Partial placenta previa:* The placenta partially covers the internal cervical os.
  3. *Marginal:* Edge of the placenta within 2 cm of the edge of the internal cervical os.
- Diagnosis
    - Transabdominal or transvaginal ultrasound (95% accurate)
  - *If the ultrasound is inconclusive:* Take the patient to the operating room and prep for a C-section. Do speculum exam: If there is local bleeding, do a C-section; if not, palpate fornices to determine if placenta is covering the os.
- *Risk factors:* Chronic hypertension, multiparity, multiple gestation, older age, previous C-sections, tobacco use, past D and C.

- Management:
  - *For preterm:* If there is no pressing need for delivery, monitor in hospital or send home after bleeding has ceased. Give transfusion to replace blood loss and tocolytics to prolong labor to 36 weeks if necessary. Even after the bleeding has stopped, repeated small hemorrhages may cause IUGR.
  - *For patients >36 weeks, those in labor or with severe hemorrhage:* perform C-section.

PLACENTAL ABRUPTION

- Placental abruption is separation of placenta from uterine wall before delivery. Presents with painful vaginal bleeding.
- *Risk factors:* Chronic hypertension, multiparity, pre-eclampsia, previous abruption, short umbilical cord, sudden decompression of an over distended uterus, thrombophilias, uterine fibroids, trauma (blunt or sudden deceleration), drugs (tobacco, cocaine or methamphetamines).
- Presents as painful vaginal bleeding (maternal and fetal blood present), hypertonic uterus, evidence of fetal distress and maternal shock.
- *Diagnosis:* Ultrasound may show retroplacental hematoma, thickening of placenta or irregular placental edge.
- *Treatment:* Correct shock (packed RBCs, fresh frozen plasma, cryoprecipitate, platelets). Manage expectantly: Close observation of mother and fetus with a low threshold to intervene if either show signs of distress.
  - If there is fetal distress, perform an emergent C-section. Fetal death can occur rapidly and delivery should occur within 20 minutes of the decision to deliver by C-section.

- Beware, fetal death may lead to coagulopathy and DIC.

UTERINE RUPTURE

- When the uterus is torn through all of its layers. It presents with cessation of contractions, recession of fetal presenting part, sudden fetal heart rate decelerations or loss of fetal heart tones. Patient may have increased pain but this may not be recognized due to epidural/narcotic medications.
- *Risk factors:* Abnormal placentation, history of uterine surgery, uterine anomalies, trauma, trial of labor after C-section, maternal connective tissue disease.
- *Management:* If the fetus is distressed, maternal position change, give IV fluids and oxygen, stop Oxytocin. Deliver immediately by emergent C-section or operative vaginal delivery. After delivery, abdominal hysterectomy is often necessary.

VASA PREVIA

- When the fetal blood vessels pass over the internal os unprotected by the placenta, they are susceptible to rupture and bleeding.
- *Presentation:* Rapid vaginal bleeding from fetoplacental circulation resulting in fetal distress. Seen as sinusoidal variation of fetal heart rate. Must recognize this pattern, as there is little time.
- *Risk factors:* Low-lying placenta, placenta previa, marginal cord insertion, multiple gestation, bilobed placentas, fetal anomalies, hx of *in vitro* fertilization.

- *Management:* Perform an emergent C-section as the fetal blood volume is only 250 mL and prepare for neonatal resuscitation with 10–20 cc/kg bolus of NS.

FETAL DEMISE

- Death prior to complete expulsion or extraction from the mother, regardless of the duration of pregnancy. Autopsy is used to identify the cause of fetal death.
- Common causes
  - *First trimester (1-14 weeks):* Fetal chromosomal abnormalities, environmental toxins, maternal anatomic defects, and endocrine factors.
  - *Second trimester (14-28 weeks):* Anatomic defects of the uterus, cervix or placenta, erythroblastosis fetalis.
  - *Third trimester (28 weeks to term):* Placental pathological conditions (circumvallate placentation, placenta previa, abruptio placentae).
  - *At any time:* Trauma, cord entanglement, anticardiolipin antibodies, infection.
- Consumptive coagulopathy (DIC) is an inappropriate activation of coagulation cascade.
  - Dead fetus produces thromboplastin, consumes platelets and factors, with fibrin deposition in small vessels causing occlusion (mix of bleeding and clotting)
  - *Occurs with:* Fetal demise, amniotic fluid embolus, pre-eclampsia and placental abruption
  - *Diagnosis:* Multiple bleeding points with purpura and petechiae
  - Labs show thrombocytopenia, hypofibrinogenemia, elevated prothrombin time, and increased fibrin split products

- *Management:* Supportive therapy to correct/prevent shock, acidosis, and tissue ischemia and prompt termination of pregnancy (correct the underlying cause).

INDUCED ABORTION

- Termination of pregnancy before fetal viability; legal definition of viability varies.
- Abortion may not be denied in first 3 months of pregnancy in any state.
- *Types:* Elective voluntary (by request of the mother); therapeutic (for the health of the mother).
- Indications for therapeutic abortions
  - *Maternal:* Cardiovascular disease, genetic syndrome (e.g. Marfan's), hematologic disease (e.g. TTP), metabolic (e.g. proliferative diabetic retinopathy), neoplastic (e.g. cervical cancer; mother needs prompt chemotherapy), neurologic (e.g. Berry aneurysm; cerebrovascular malformation), renal disease, intrauterine infection, severe pre-eclampsia/eclampsia.
  - *Fetal indications:* Major malformation (anencephaly), genetic (Tay–Sachs disease).
- Work-up
  - *Physical assessment:* Ultrasound if uterine size and dates do not match
  - *Maternal blood and Rh type:* If Rh negative, give RhoGAM prophylactically
  - Patient counseling should be performed prior to any abortion.

ABORTION METHODS

Medical

- Before 9 weeks gestation:
  - Antiprogesterones such as Mifepristone (RU 486) or epostane. Without progesterone, the uterine lining sloughs off.
  - Methotrexate IM + intrauterine Misoprostol 1 week later. Methotrexate is a folic acid antagonist that interferes with cell division.
- *Up to 20 weeks:* Intravaginal prostaglandin E2 or PGF2α with urea.

Surgical

- *First trimester:* Cervical dilation followed by aspiration curettage (D&C): Risks include cervical/uterine injury and Asherman's syndrome.
- *Second trimester* dilation and evacuation. Risks include infection, incomplete removal of products of conception (POC), disseminated intravascular coagulation (DIC), bleeding, cervical laceration, uterine perforation/rupture, psychological sequelae, death.
- Rarely used methods of abortion, are methods of last resort: Surgical: hysterotomy (C-section of a preterm fetus) or hysterectomy.

MEDICATIONS IN PREGNANCY

- General:
  - Lipid-soluble substances readily cross the placenta. Water-soluble substances cross less well because of their larger molecular weight. Drugs bound to plasma proteins do not cross very freely. The minimal effective dose of all meds should be used.
- Vitamin A in doses >25,000 IU/day, and in medications like Accutane has a risk of craniofacial, cardiac, thymic, and CNS anomalies.
- Methotrexate and Aminopterin (folic acid derivatives), as well as Phenytoin (decreases folic acid absorption) cause IUGR, mental retardation, and craniofacial malformations.
- Warfarin crosses the placenta and is associated with chondrodysplasia punctata, likely due to microhemorrhages during development. Heparin and LMWH have large negative charges and do not cross the placenta.
- Insulin is safe in pregnancy as it is large and does not cross placenta. Effect of oral hypoglycemic agents is unknown.
- Psychiatric medications:
  - Valproic acid and Carbamazepine have a 1% risk of neural tube defects.
  - Imipramine (Tofranil) is associated with fetal cardiac anomalies. Chlordiazepoxide (Librium) is associated with congenital anomalies, but Paxil (Fluoxetine) is not associated.
  - Diazepam is associated with fetal hypothermia, hypotonia, and respiratory depression.

Pregnancy Complications

ANTIBIOTICS, ANDROGENS AND PAIN MEDICATIONS

- Pain medications:
  - Aspirin does not have teratogenic effects when taken early, but when taken near delivery can decrease uterine contractility, delay onset of labor, prolong the duration of labor and carry an increased risk of maternal bleeding.
  - Ibuprofen (Motrin, Advil) and Naproxen (Naprosyn) have not shown fetal effects with short-term use, however, long-term use may lead to oligohydramnios and constriction of the fetal ductus arteriosus.
  - Acetaminophen (Tylenol, Datril) has shown no evidence of teratogenicity.
- Antibiotics:
  - Penicillin, Cephalosporin, and Erythromycin are safe, Doxycycline has no risk in T1.
  - Aminoglycosides (Streptomycin) carry a risk of deafness.
  - Trimethoprim in first trimester is associated with an increased risk of birth defects.
  - Tetracycline inhibits bone growth, bind to developing enamel and discolor the teeth. Quinolones (Ciprofloxacin, Norfloxacin) have a high affinity for cartilage and bone tissue and may cause arthropathies in children.
- Androgens/Progestins:
  - Androgens may masculinize a developing female fetus
  - Progestins (Danazol) may cause clitoromegaly and labial fusion if given prior to 13 weeks gestation.

ASTHMATIC AND CARDIOVASCULAR MEDICATIONS

- Antiasthmatics:
  - Epinephrine exposure after T1 has been associated with minor malformations.
  - Terbutaline (Brethine) is not associated with birth defects but long-term use is associated with increased risk of glucose intolerance.
  - Isoproterenol (Isuprel) and Albuterol (Ventolin) are not teratogenic.
  - Corticosteroids are inactivated by the placenta when given to the mother so that <10% of maternal dose gets to the fetus.
- Cardiovascular:
  - Angiotensin-converting enzyme inhibitors (Vasotec, Capoten) can cause fetal renal tubular dysplasia in second and third trimester, leading to oligohydramnios, fetal limb contractures, craniofacial deformities, hypoplastic lung development.
  - Propranolol (Inderal) shows no evidence of teratogenicity: Fetal bradycardia has been seen as a direct dose effect and there is an increased risk of IUGR with maternal use.

BIBLIOGRAPHY

ACOG Practice Bulletin No. 102: management of stillbirth. Obstet Gynecol. 2009;113:748.

American College of Obstetric Committee on Obstetric Practice. Committee Opinion no. 514: emergent therapy for acute-onset, severe hypertension with Pre-eclampsia or eclampsia. Obstet Gynecol. 2011;118:1465.

American College of Obstetricians and Gynecologists. ACOG Practice Bulletin. Clinical management guidelines for obstetrician-gynecologists. Number 37, August 2002. (Replaces Practice Bulletin Number 32, November 2001). Thyroid disease in pregnancy. Obstet Gynecol. 2002;100:387.

American College of Obstetricians and Gynecologists. Diagnosis and management of Pre-eclampsia and eclampsia. ACOG practice bulletin #33. American College of Obstetricians and Gynecologists, Washington, DC 2002. Obstet Gynecol. 2002.

American College of Obstetricians and Gynecologists. Induction of labor with misoprostol. ACOG Committee Opinioin #228, American College of Obstetricians and Gynecologists, Washington, DC 2000.

American College of Obstetricians and Gynecologists. Practice bulletin no. 137: Gestational diabetes mellitus. Obstet Gynecol. 2013;122:406.

American Diabetes Association. Standards of medical care in diabetes 2013. Diabetes Care. 2013;36 (Suppl 1):S11.

Ansari AA, Fett JD, Carraway RE, et al. Autoimmune mechanisms as the basis for human peripartum cardiomyopathy. Clin Rev Allergy Immunol. 2002;23:301.

Arya R. How I manage venous thromboembolism in pregnancy. Br J Haematol. 2011;153:698.

Bahar A, Abusham A, Eskandar M, et al. Risk factors and pregnancy outcome in different types of placenta previa. J Obstet Gynaecol Can. 2009;31:126.

Barton JR, O'brien JM, Bergauer NK, et al. Mild gestational hypertension remote from term: progression and outcome. Am J Obstet Gynecol. 2001;184:979.

Baschat AA. Fetal growth restriction—from observation to intervention. J Perinat Med. 2010;38:239.

Batalle D, et al. Altered small-world topology of structural brain networks in infants with intrauterine growth restriction and its association with later neurodevelopmental outcome. Neuro Image. 2012;60(2):1352-66.

Bates SM, Ginsberg JS. How we manage venous thromboembolism during pregnancy. Blood. 2002;100:3470.

Bates SM, Greer IA, Middeldorp S, et al. VTE, thrombophilia, antithrombotic therapy, and pregnancy: Antithrombotic Therapy and Prevention of Thrombosis, 9th edn: American College of Chest Physicians Evidence-Based Clinical Practice Guidelines. Chest. 2012; 141:e691S.

Benedetto C, Marozio L, Tancredi A, et al. Biochemistry of HELLP syndrome. Adv Clin Chem. 2011;53:85.

Berghella V, Baxter JK, Chauhan SP. Evidence-based labor and delivery management. Am J Obstet Gynecol. 2008;199:445.

Bryant AG, Grimes DA, Garrett JM, Stuart GS. Second-trimester abortion for fetal anomalies or fetal death: labor induction compared with dilation and evacuation. Obstet Gynecol. 2011;117:788.

Casey BM, Dashe JS, Wells CE, et al. Subclinical hyperthyroidism and pregnancy outcomes. Obstet Gynecol. 2006;107:337.

Cepni I, Ocal P, Erkan S, Erzik B. Conservative treatment of cervical ectopic pregnancy with transvaginal ultrasound-guided aspiration and single-dose methotrexate. Fertil Steril. 2004;81:1130.

Chen YH, Keller J, Lin CC, et al. Pneumonia and pregnancy outcomes: a nationwide population-based study. Am J Obstet Gynecol. 2012;207:288.e1.

Chibber R, El-Saleh E, Al Fadhli R, et al. Uterine rupture and subsequent pregnancy outcome--how safe is it? A 25-year study. J Matern Fetal Neonatal Med. 2010;23:421.

Cowett AA, Golub RM, Grobman WA. Cost-effectiveness of dilation and evacuation versus the induction of labor for second-trimester pregnancy termination. Am J Obstet Gynecol. 2006;194:768.

Cruz MO, Gao W, Hibbard JU. What is the optimal time for delivery in women with gestational hypertension? Am J Obstet Gynecol. 2012;207:214.e1.

Dhulkotia JS, Ola B, Fraser R, Farrell T. Oral hypoglycemic agents vs insulin in management of gestational diabetes: a systematic review and metaanalysis. Am J Obstet Gynecol. 2010;203:457.e1.

Dombrowski MP, Schatz M. ACOG Committee on Practice Bulletins-Obstetrics. ACOG practice bulletin: clinical management guidelines for obstetrician-gynecologists number 90, February 2008: asthma in pregnancy. Obstet Gynecol. 2008;111:457.

Dover RW, Powell MC. Management of a primary abdominal pregnancy. Am J Obstet Gynecol. 1995;172:1603.

Edlow AG, Hou MY, Maurer R, et al. Uterine evacuation for second-trimester fetal death and maternal morbidity. Obstet Gynecol. 2011;117:307.

EURAP Study Group. Seizure control and treatment in pregnancy: observations from the EURAP epilepsy pregnancy registry. Neurology. 2006;66:354.

Feldkamp ML, Meyer RE, Krikov S, Botto LD. Acetaminophen use in pregnancy and risk of birth defects: findings from the National Birth Defects Prevention Study. Obstet Gynecol. 2010;115:109.

Fett JD, Christie LG, Carraway RD, Murphy JG. Five-year prospective study of the incidence and prognosis of peripartum cardiomyopathy at a single institution. Mayo Clin Proc. 2005;80:1602.

Gagnon R, Morin L, Bly S, et al. Guidelines for the management of vasa previa. J Obstet Gynaecol Can. 2009;31:748.

Gilo NB, Amini D, Landy HJ. Appendicitis and cholecystitis in pregnancy. Clin Obstet Gynecol. 2009;52:586.

Guise JM, Denman MA, Emeis C, et al. Vaginal birth after cesarean: new insights on maternal and neonatal outcomes. Obstet Gynecol. 2010;115:1267.

Heinonen OP, Slone D, Shapiro S. Birth defects and drugs in pregnancy, PSG Publishing, Littleton, MA, 1977.

Icians and Gynecologists. ACOG committee opinion no. 560: Medically indicated late-preterm and early-term deliveries. Obstet Gynecol. 2013;121:908.

Jebbink J, Wolters A, Fernando F, et al. Molecular genetics of Pre-eclampsia and HELLP syndrome - a review. Biochim Biophys Acta 2012;1822:1960.

Kaplan JE, Benson C, Holmes KK, et al. Guidelines for prevention and treatment of opportunistic infections in HIV-infected adults and adolescents: recommendations from CDC, the National Institutes of Health, and the HIV Medicine Association of the Infectious Diseases Society of America. MMWR Recomm Rep. 2009;58:1.

Koopmans CM, Bijlenga D, Groen H, et al. Induction of labour versus expectant monitoring for gestational hypertension or mild pre-eclampsia after 36 weeks' gestation (HYPITAT): a multicentre, open-label randomised controlled trial. Lancet. 2009;374:979.

Krassas GE, Poppe K, Glinoer D. Thyroid function and human reproductive health. Endocr Rev. 2010;31:702.

Kupesic Plavsic S, et al. Pregnancy Loss and Pregnancy Complications. Video Atlas of Clinical Skills in Ob Gyn. New Delhi: Jaypee Publisher, 2012.

Kweder SL. Drugs and biologics in pregnancy and breastfeeding: FDA in the 21st century. Birth Defects Res A Clin Mol Teratol. 2008;82:605.

Le J, Briggs GG, McKeown A, Bustillo G. Urinary tract infections during pregnancy. Ann Pharmacother. 2004;38:1692.

Lurie S, Feinstein M, Mamet Y. Disseminated intravascular coagulopathy in pregnancy: thorough comprehension of etiology and management reduces obstetricians› stress. Arch Gynecol Obstet. 2000;263:126.

Magann EF, Chauhan SP, Bofill JA, et al. Maternal morbidity and mortality associated with intrauterine fetal demise: five-year experience in a tertiary referral hospital. South Med. J 2001;94:493.

McCormack RA, Doherty DA, Magann EF, et al. Antepartum bleeding of unknown origin in the second half of pregnancy and pregnancy outcomes. BJOG. 2008;115:1451.

McPherson JA, Odibo AO, Shanks AL, et al. Adverse outcomes in twin pregnancies complicated by early vaginal bleeding. Am J Obstet Gynecol. 2013;208:56.e1.

Melamed N, Aviram A, Silver M, et al. Pregnancy course and outcome following blunt trauma. J Matern Fetal Neonatal Med. 2012;25:1612.

Muench MV, Baschat AA, Reddy UM, et al. Kleihauer-betke testing is important in all cases of maternal trauma. J Trauma. 2004;57:1094.

Oppenheimer L. Society of Obstetricians and Gynaecologists of Canada. Diagnosis and management of placenta previa. J Obstet Gynaecol Can. 2007;29:261.

Perritt JB, Burke A, Edelman AB. Interruption of nonviable pregnancies of 24-28 weeks, gestation using medical methods: release date June 2013 SFP guideline #20133. Contraception. 2013;88:341.

Petitti, DB. Perinatal epidemiology: Studying the effects of illness and medications during pregnancy. Immunol Allergy Clin North Am. 2000;20:673.

Ramin KD, Ramsey PS. Disease of the gallbladder and pancreas in pregnancy. Obstet Gynecol Clin North Am. 2001;28:571.

Rausch ME, Barnhart KT. Serum biomarkers for detecting ectopic pregnancy. Clin Obstet Gynecol. 2012;55:418.

Redline RW. Placental pathology: a systematic approach with clinical correlations. Placenta. 2008;29 (Suppl A):S86.

Sheiner E, Shoham-Vardi I, Hallak M, et al. Placenta previa: obstetric risk factors and pregnancy outcome. J Matern Fetal Med. 2001;10:414.

Shotan A, Ostrzega E, Mehra A, et al. Incidence of arrhythmias in normal pregnancy and relation to palpitations, dizziness, and syncope. Am J Cardiol. 1997;79:1061.

Sibai BM. Diagnosis, controversies, and management of the syndrome of hemolysis, elevated liver enzymes, and low platelet count. Obstet Gynecol. 2004;103:981.

Silva C, Sammel MD, Zhou L, et al. Human chorionic gonadotropin profile for women with ectopic pregnancy. Obstet Gynecol. 2006;107:605.

Sir-Petermann T, Maliqueo M, Angel B, et al. Maternal serum androgens in pregnant women with polycystic ovarian syndrome: possible implications in prenatal androgenization. Hum Reprod. 2002;17:2573.

Society for Maternal-Fetal Medicine Publications Committee, Berkley E, Chauhan SP, Abuhamad A. Doppler assessment of the fetus with intrauterine growth restriction. Am J Obstet Gynecol. 2012.

Stubblefield PG, Carr-Ellis S, Borgatta L. Methods for induced abortion. Obstet Gynecol. 2004;104:174.

Task Force on the Management of Cardiovascular Diseases During Pregnancy of the European Society of Cardiology. Expert consensus document on management of cardiovascular diseases during pregnancy. Eur Heart J. 2003;24:761.

Thurmond A, Mendelson E, Böhm-Vélez M, et al. Role of imaging in second and third trimester bleeding. American College of Radiology. ACR Appropriateness Criteria. Radiology. 2000;215 (Suppl):895.

Tikkanen M. Placental abruption: epidemiology, risk factors and consequences. Acta Obstet Gynecol Scand. 2011;90:140.

Tomson T, Perucca E, Battino D. Navigating toward fetal and maternal health: the challenge of treating epilepsy in pregnancy. Epilepsia. 2004;45:1171.

Towers CV, Burkhart AE. Pregnancy outcome after a primary antenatal hemorrhage between 16 and 24 weeks' gestation. Am J Obstet Gynecol. 2008;198:684.e1.

Undergraduate Medical Education Committee (UMEC) of the Association of Professors of Gynecology and Obstetrics (APGO). The Ob-gyn Clerkship: Your Guide to Success. 2006.

Veille JC. Peripartum cardiomyopathies: a review. Am J Obstet Gynecol. 1984;148:805.

Velez Edwards DR, Baird DD, Hasan R, et al. First-trimester bleeding characteristics associate with increased risk of preterm birth: data from a prospective pregnancy cohort. Hum Reprod. 2012;27:54.

Visintin C, Mugglestone MA, Almerie MQ, et al. Management of hypertensive disorders during pregnancy: summary of NICE guidance. BMJ. 2010;341:c2207.

Walker SP, Permezel M, Berkovic SF. The management of epilepsy in pregnancy. BJOG. 2009;116:758.

Working group report on high blood pressure in pregnancy. National Institutes of Health, Washington, DC 2000.

3
Labor and Delivery

CHAPTER OUTLINES

- Labor Progress, Vaginal Delivery Notes
- Assessing a Patient in Labor
- Rupture of Membranes
- Vaginal Examinations
- Digital Cervical Examination
- Labor Pain Control
- Stages of Labor
- Labor Movements
- Postpartum Note

LABOR PROGRESS, VAGINAL DELIVERY NOTES

Labor Admission and Progress Notes

S: Comfortable (Y/N), epidural (Y/N), complaints (e.g. leakage of fluid, vaginal bleeding, contractions, etc.) in _____ stage of labor.

HPI: _ yo G_P__ @ ___ weeks by LMP consistent with 1st trimester US (or by US alone) presents for _____. Patient reports +/–FM, LOF, VB, or contractions (Y/N). +/– HA, vision changes, RUQ pain. Pregnancy complicated by _____. Prenatal care @ _____.

LMP: _____

EDD: _____

OB Hx: G_P____ (T- term, P- preterm, A- abortions, L-living children); mention all deliveries (year; term or preterm, if preterm - why; vaginal or cesarean delivery, type of cesarean and why; male of female; weight; complications.

Abortions: SAB (spontaneous) vs. EAB (elective), note GA and if D&C performed).

GYN Hx: h/o STDs, abnormal Paps, etc.

*PMH (past medical history):*_____

PSH (past surgical history): For example, D&C___, appendectomy

Meds: _____

Allergies: _____ (always note reaction, e.g. PCL rash)

Family Hx: Mother___, Father___ (DM, HTN). +/- birth defects, mental retardation, bleeding or clotting disorders

Social Hx: +/- tobacco, EtOH, drugs. Living situation. Occupation. Feels safe? +/- Depression.

ROS

- *Gen:* +/- Fever/chills
- *HEENT:* Vision changes, sore throat, rhinorrhea
- *CV:* Palpitations, chest pain
- *Pulm:* SOB, prolonged cough
- *GI:* Abdominal pain, nausea, vomiting, diarrhea, constipation
- *GU:* Dysuria, hematuria, frequency, abnormal vaginal discharge
- *MS:* Joint pain, swelling

- *Neuro:* Severe headache, weakness
- *Heme:* h/o anemia or blood clots
- *Psych:* Depression or anxiety
- *Physical exam:*
- *VS:* BP___, HR __, RR __, O_2 Sat __
- *FHT (baby's vitals):* Baseline, variability (absent, minimal, moderate, marked), accelerations, decelerations (state type-early, late, variable)
- *Toco:* q 5 minutes (or 2 in 1 hour, or none)
- *Gen:* A/O (alert and oriented), NAD (no acute distress) or appears uncomfortable, etc.
- *CV:* RRR (regular rate and rhythm), + SEM (systolic ejection murmur)
- *Pulm:* CTAB (clear to auscultation bilaterally)
- *Abd:* 'gravid' Fundal Height = ___cm. EFW (estimated fetal weight)__ kg/lbs. Leopolds = presentation
- *Ext:* +/– edema, calves (tender, nontender)
- *Neuro:* DTRs (deep tendon reflexes) ___, clonus Y/N *(needed if any concern about pre-eclampsia)*
- *SSE (sterile speculum exam):* No bleeding or pooling; cervix visually dilated to ___cm

SVE (sterile vaginal exam): Cervix (dilatation, e.g. 3 cm)/effacement (in %, e.g. 50%), membranes (intact, rupture of membranes, ROM time), station (e.g. -1)

- *Wet Prep:* +/– yeast, clue cells, or trich. Nitrazine and Ferning +/–
- *Urine Dip:* +/–

- *PNL (prenatal labs):* BG/Rh/HIV/HepB/RPR/GC (gonorrhea/chlamydia)/CF (cystic fibrosis)/Hgb/glucose tolerance test/GBS status

(e.g. O+/Ab-/HIV-/HepB-/RPR NR /CF-/GC-/Hgb 13.2/Pap NIL (negative for intraepithelial lesion/1 hour 72/GBS- (GBS negative)
- *GBS +:* Antibiotics (Y/N)
- *Premature labor:* Steroids given (Y/N)
- *Level II US:* EFW ___ g (__%), presentation, 3VC (Y/N), placenta (anterior, posterior, etc.), normal/abnormal fetal anatomy, BPP (biophysical profile)__ , Doppler __
- *FWB (fetal wellbeing) reassuring:* FHT (fetal heart tracing category)
    - Admit to L&D, anticipate vaginal delivery
    - NPO, IVF (nothing per os/intravenous fluids).

Vaginal Delivery Note

- NSVD of viable (male/female) infant over an intact perineum @ (time)
- Apgars _&_, wt __g. Position (e.g. LOA), bulb suction, (nuchal cord × ?, reducible).
- Spontaneous delivery of intact 3-vessel cord placenta @ (time), fundal massage and Pitocin initiated, fundus firm.
- __-degree perineal laceration repaired under local anesthesia with __-0 vicryl.
- Estimated blood loss (EBL) = ___ cc. Mom and baby stable Y/N). Doctors were ___

ASSESSING A PATIENT IN LABOR

- *False labor (Braxton Hicks contractions):* Irregular contractions, same intensity throughout, cervix not dilated, discomfort relieved by medications.
- *True labor:* Regular contractions with increase in intensity and dilated cervix. Signs are bloody show, rupture of membranes (diagnose by Nitrazine, Fern Tests).
- Maternal blood pressure and pulse should be evaluated and recorded every 10 minutes. Oral intake is limited to small sips of water, ice chips, or hard candies.
    - *If no prenatal care check:* CBC, blood group and Rh typing, rapid HIV, urine testing.
    - *Those with prenatal care require:* Urine test for protein or glucose, CBC, blood for cross matching.
- Always obtain from a laboring patient:
    - Time of onset and frequency of contractions, rupture membranes, presence of vaginal bleeding, regularity of fetal activity, last food intake, use of medications, allergies to medications. Determine if high- or low-risk pregnancy.
- Monitor uterine contractions by internal or external uterine pressure monitors. Pressure is calculated by increases in uterine pressure above baseline (8–12 mm Hg) multiplied by frequency of contractions per 10 minutes.
    - Uterine contractions in the first stage of labor increase progressively in intensity from 25 mm Hg to 50 mm Hg, and the frequency increases from three to five contractions per 10 minutes.

- Contractions in the second stage increase further (aided by maternal bearing down) to 80–100 mm Hg, and the frequency increases to 5–6 per 10 minutes.

RUPTURE OF MEMBRANES

- A digital examination should not be performed, as it increases the risk of infection:
    - *Sterile speculum examination (SSE):* Visualize extent of cervical effacement and dilation, and exclude prolapsed cord or protruding fetal extremity.
    - *Pool test:* Identify fluid coming from the cervix or pooled in the posterior fornix of the vagina → supports diagnosis of PROM.
    - *Nitrazine test (NT):* Put fluid on nitrazine paper, which turns blue if fluid is alkaline. Alkaline pH indicates fluid is amniotic.
    - *Ferning test:* A swab from the posterior fornix is smeared on a slide, allowed to dry, and examined under a microscope for "ferning" → + for amniotic fluid.
- *ROM:* Rupture of membranes.
- *PROM:* Premature rupture of membranes (ROM before the onset of labor).
- *PPROM:* Preterm (<37 weeks) premature rupture of membranes
    - If <24 weeks, increased risk of oligohydramnios that may cause pulmonary hypoplasia.
    - Increased risk of premature birth.

- *Prolonged rupture of membranes:* Membranes ruptured >18 hours before delivery
  - Increased risk of chorioamnionitis, neonatal infection and umbilical cord prolapse.
  - *Etiology:* Unknown but hypothesized—vaginal and cervical infections, incompetent cervix, abnormal membranes, and nutritional deficiencies.

VAGINAL EXAMINATIONS

- Vaginal examinations should be kept to the minimum required for the evaluation of a normal labor pattern, for example, every 4 hours in latent phase and every 2 hours in active phase. Sterile gloves and lubricant should be utilized.
- Perform a sterile speculum examination prior to a digital examination if you suspect rupture of membranes, preterm labor or placenta previa. Otherwise, a digital cervical examination may be performed.
- To assess vaginal fluid to determine if membranes have already ruptured:
  - Use a sterile speculum to assess fluid in the posterior vaginal fornix (pool test).
  - Fluid may be collected on a swab if the source of fluid is unclear:
    - *Ferning test* (high estrogen content of amniotic fluid causes fern pattern on slide when air dried). Confirms ROM in 85–98% of cases.

- *Nitrazine test:* Nitrazine paper is pH sensitive and turns blue with amniotic fluid as it is more alkaline than vaginal secretions (pH = 7.15) 90–98% accurate.
- Fluid should also be examined for vernix or meconium.
    - The presence of meconium in the amniotic fluid may indicate fetal distress. Meconium staining more common in term and post-term pregnancies than preterm.
    - Meconium aspiration syndrome is seen as infant tachypnea, costal retractions, cyanosis, coarse breath sounds.

DIGITAL CERVICAL EXAMINATION

- Effacement describes the length of the cervix which usually thins and softens in labor. The normal length is 3–4 cm. 50% is around 2 cm length. When the cervix becomes as thin as the areas surrounding the cervix, it is 100% effaced.
    - Palpate with finger and estimate the length from the internal to external os.
- Dilation is the size of the opening of the cervix. Ranges from closed (zero) to fully dilated (10 cm).
    - Sweep a finger from the margin of the cervix on one side to the opposite side.
- Cervical position describes the location of cervix with respect to the fetal presenting part, usually progresses from posterior to anterior during labor.

- *Posterior:* Difficult to palpate because it is behind the fetus, and high in the pelvis.
- *Anterior:* Easy to palpate, low down in pelvis.
- Cervical consistency ranges from firm to soft. Soft is favorable for labor.
- *Bishop score* rates if cervix is ready for delivery. If sum >8 is a favorable cervix
  - *1 pt:* Dilated 1–2 cm, effaced 40–50%, station -2, cervix mid position, medium consistency.
  - *2 pt:* Dilated 3–4 cm, effaced 60–70%, station -1 or 0, cervix anterior position, soft consistency.
  - *3 pt:* Dilated 5–6 cm, effaced >80%, station >+1, +2.
- Cervical ripening agents
  - Cervidil (prostaglandin E2/dinoprostone) 10 mg. Insert q 12 hours, maximum 3 doses.
  - Cytotec (prostaglandin E1/misoprostol) 25 mcg (1/4 of 100 mcg pill) vaginally q 4 hours.
  - Oxytocin.

LABOR PAIN CONTROL

- Innervation:
  - Early labor pain is from uterine contractions. Visceral sensory fibers from the uterus, cervix, and upper vagina run with T11-12 and L1.
  - Second stage of labor pain is from genital tract, along the pudendal nerve S2-4.
- Nonpharmacological methods of pain control:

- Appropriate antepartum training in breathing. Psychological support (friend or family member). Considerate physicians and labor assistants (doulas) who instill confidence.
- Pain relief with a narcotic (Meperidine/Stadol/Fentanyl/Nalbuphine) plus an antiemetic (Promethazine) is both safe and effective.
  - Slight, bearable discomfort should still be felt at the height of a contraction.
  - *Phenergan + Meperidine IM:* Analgesia peak at 45 minutes. IV—effects are immediate.
  - *Naloxone hydrochloride:* Displaces the narcotic from receptors in the CNS. 0.1 mg/kg of body weight of the newborn injected into the umbilical vein and acts in 2 minutes.
- General anesthesia should be given as late as possible to minimize newborn respiratory depression. All anesthetic agents that depress the maternal CNS cross the placenta and depress the fetal CNS.
- Epidural anesthesia relieves pain of uterine contractions
  - *Lumbar block:* Abdominal delivery (T8-S1) or Caudal block vaginal delivery (T10-S5).
  - Risks of accidental spinal block, hypotension, convulsions, prolongation of labor.

STAGES OF LABOR

- *First stage* begins with onset of labor (uterine contractions of sufficient frequency, intensity, and duration to result in

effacement and dilation of the cervix), and ends when the cervix is fully/completely dilated to 10 cm. Two phases:
- *Latent phase:* From onset of labor to 4 cm dilatation. Lasts 20 hours in nulliparous, 14 hours in multiparous.
- *Active phase:* Rapid dilation from 4 to 10 cm dilation, takes nulliparous 1.2 cm/h, multiparous 1.5 cm/h. Fetal descent at 7–8 cm.

- *Second stage* begins with a fully dilated cervix and ends with delivery of the fetus.
    - Fetus descends in nulliparous women 1 cm/h, multiparous at 2 cm/h.
    - The modified Ritgen maneuver presents the smallest diameter for delivery. Place one hand over the perineum with upward pressure on the fetal chin, other hand pressing down on the fetal occiput during a contraction.
    - After delivery of the head, check for a nuchal cord by passing a finger along the neck. If felt remove with finger over the infant's head, unless tight, then clamp and cut.
    - Shoulders normally deliver spontaneously, grasp sides of head with both hands, gentle downward traction applied until anterior shoulder descends under the pubic arch, then upward traction to deliver posterior shoulder.
    - Typically, the rest of the body rapidly follows the delivery of the shoulders.

- *Third stage* is placental separation. Usually <10 minutes, prolonged if >30 minutes.

- Three signs are: Gush of blood, lengthening umbilical cord, uterine fundus firming.

LABOR MOVEMENTS

Cardinal movements are changes in the position of the fetal head during birth.

- *Engagement* is the descent of the biparietal diameter to the plane of the pelvic inlet (0 station). Often occurs before the onset of true labor, especially in nulliparous women.
- *Descent* is the fetal head passing down into the pelvis. It occurs in a discontinuous fashion. The greatest rate of descent occurs in the deceleration phase of the first stage of labor and during the second stage of labor.
- *Flexion* refers to the chin-to-chest position that the fetus takes to present the smallest possible diameter of the fetal head to the birth canal.
- *Internal rotation* refers to the fetal occiput gradually rotating toward the pubic symphysis.
- *Extension* occurs after the fetus has descended to the maternal vulva. This brings the base of the occiput into contact with the inferior margin of the symphysis pubis, where the birth canal curves upward. The fetal head is delivered by extension from the flexed to the extended position, curving under and past the pubic symphysis.
- *External rotation:* The fetus resumes its normal "face-forward" position with the occiput and spine in the same plane. External rotation is completed by rotation of the

fetal body to the transverse position (one shoulder anterior behind the pubic symphysis and one posterior).
- *Expulsion:* Further descent brings the anterior shoulder to the level of the pubic symphysis. The shoulder is delivered under the pubic symphysis and then the rest of the body is quickly delivered.

POSTPARTUM NOTE

- *S:* __ yo; G__P__ postpartum day#____ S/P NSVD/LTCS/VBAC/RCS. Pain controlled? Tolerating diet without nausea/vomiting? Ambulating with/without dizziness? Denies or reports chest pain/shortness of breath/calf pain?
- *Ask about "B's":* Bleeding (lochia amount and color), Blues (depression), Bowel (BM or flatus), Bladder (voiding >30 cc/h), breast (feeding and pain), baby (boy/girl in room or in nursery/NICU, ask about circumcision for male infant), Birth control wishes.
- *O:* Vital signs (BP, P, RR, body temperature), intake and output.
- *PE:* Include fundal assessment, incision status.
- *Labs:* Including H/H.

  A/P: __ yo G_P__ postpartum day#_ S/P NSVD/1LTCS/VBAC/RCS.
  - Pain controlled with Motrin and Darvocet.
  - Advance diet to general (clears, full liquid, etc.) as tolerated (patient after CS).
  - Urine output appropriate. Discontinue Foley catheter (patients after CS).
  - Encourage ambulation (patients after CS).

- Sequential compression devices for DVT prophylaxis (patients after CS).
- For patients with constipation, prescribe Colace. For issues with gas, use Simethicone.
- For postoperative anemia prescribe iron.
- For breastfeeding patients recommend multivitamins.
- Rhogam prior to discharge for Rh negative patients. For rubella nonimmune patients, give MMR prior to discharge.
- For male infants, discuss desire for circumcision.

BIBLIOGRAPHY

Bailit JL, Dierker L, Blanchard MH, Mercer BM. Outcomes of women presenting in active versus latent phase of spontaneous labor. Obstet Gynecol 2005;105:77.

Berghella V, Baxter JK, Chauhan SP. Evidence-based labor and delivery management. Am J Obstet Gynecol 2008;199:445.

Cheng YW, Delaney SS, Hopkins LM, Caughey AB. The association between the length of first stage of labor, mode of delivery, and perinatal outcomes in women undergoing induction of labor. Am J Obstet Gynecol 2009;201:477.e1.

Copper RL, Goldenberg RL, Davis RO, et al. Warning symptoms, uterine contractions, and cervical examination findings in women at risk of preterm delivery. Am J Obstet Gynecol 1990;162:748.

Downe S, Gyte GM, Dahlen HG, Singata M. Routine vaginal examinations for assessing progress of labour to improve outcomes for women and babies at term. Cochrane Database Syst Rev 2013;7.

Duignan NM, Studd JW, Hughes AO. Characteristics of normal labour in different racial groups. Br J Obstet Gynaecol 1975;82:593.

Goetzl LM, ACOG Committee on Practice Bulletins-Obstetrics. ACOG Practice Bulletin. Clinical Management Guidelines for Obstetrician-Gynecologists Number 36, July 2002. Obstetric analgesia and anesthesia. Obstet Gynecol 2002;100:177.

Harper LM, Caughey AB, Odibo AO, et al. Normal progress of induced labor. Obstet Gynecol 2012;119:1113.

Herbst A, Källén K. Time between membrane rupture and delivery and septicemia in term neonates. Obstet Gynecol 2007;110:612.

Lanham M, Morgan H. University of Michigan OB Gyn Survival Guide, 2011.

Lanham M, Morgan H. University of Michigan OB-Gyn Survival Guide, 2011.

Locatelli A, Regalia AL, Patregnani C, et al. Prognostic value of change in amniotic fluid color during labor. Fetal Diagn Ther 2005;20:5.

Lockwood CJ, Dudenhausen JW. New approaches to the prediction of preterm delivery. J Perinat Med 1993;21:441.

Mattingly JE, D'Alessio J, Ramanathan J. Effects of obstetric analgesics and anesthetics on the neonate: a review. Paediatr Drugs 2003;5:615.

Mercer BM. Preterm premature ruptures of the membranes: current approaches to evaluation and management. Obstet Gynecol Clin North Am 2005;32:411.

Romero R, Hsu YC, Athanassiadis AP, et al. Preterm delivery: a risk factor for retained placenta. Am J Obstet Gynecol 1990;163:823.

Saito M, Okutomi T, Kanai Y, et al. Patient-controlled epidural analgesia during labor using ropivacaine and fentanyl provides better maternal satisfaction with less local anesthetic requirement. J Anesth 2005;19:208.

Tran SH, Cheng YW, Kaimal AJ, Caughey AB. Length of rupture of membranes in the setting of premature rupture of membranes at term and infectious maternal morbidity. Am J Obstet Gynecol 2008;198:700.e1.

Vintzileos AM. Antepartum surveillance in preterm rupture of membranes. J Perinat Med 1996;24:319.

Williams Obstetrics, 23rd Ed, Cunningham, FG, Leveno, KJ, Bloom, JC, et al (Eds), McGraw-Hill, 2010.

Zhang J, Troendle J, Mikolajczyk R, et al. The natural history of the normal first stage of labor. Obstet Gynecol 2010;115:705.

4
Abnormal Labor

CHAPTER OUTLINES

- Labor Induction
- Cesarean Section
- Preterm Labor
- Magnesium Note
- Management of Prematures Rupture of Membranes
- Labor Dystocia
- Abnormal Third Stage of Labor
- Postpartum Hemorrhage
- Shoulder Dystocia
- Breech

LABOR INDUCTION

- Do not schedule elective, nonmedically indicated inductions of labor or cesarean deliveries before 39 weeks 0 days gestational age.
  - Increased risk of learning disabilities and a potential increase in morbidity/mortality.
- Do not schedule elective, nonmedically indicated inductions of labor between 39 weeks 0 days and 41 weeks 0 days unless the cervix is deemed favorable.
  - Ideally, labor should start on its own initiative whenever possible. Higher cesarean delivery rates result from inductions of labor when the cervix is unfavorable.
- Induction is indicated when waiting for normal labor is dangerous to the mother or the fetus.

- *Maternal:* Premature ROM, diabetes mellitus, heart disease, prolonged labor, prolonged pregnancy.
- *Fetal:* IUGR, abnormal fetal testing, infection, and Rh incompatibility.
- Contraindications
  - *Maternal:* Contracted pelvis, prior uterine surgery (controversial), classic cesarean section, and history of myomectomy.
  - *Fetal:* Lung immaturity, acute distress, and abnormal presentation.
- *Oxytocin:* A synthetic hormone that stimulates uterine contractions: Acts promptly when given intravenously; should not be employed for more than few hours.
  - *Complications:* Potent antidiuretic effects of Oxytocin (Oxytocin is related structurally and functionally to vasopressin or antidiuretic hormone); can cause water intoxication, which can lead to convulsions, coma and death. Beware of the risk of uterine overstimulation.
- *Prostaglandins:* Used for cervical ripening and induction
  - *Misoprostol, a synthetic PGE1 analog:* It can be administered intravaginally or orally.
  - *PGE2 gel and vaginal insert:* Both contain dinoprostone.

CESAREAN SECTION

- Birth of a fetus through incisions in the abdominal wall and uterine wall
  - *Low transverse cesarean section (LCTS):* Incision in lower uterine segment

- *Classical:* Vertical incision in uterine corpus, done when lower uterine segment is not developed or fetus is in transverse lie with back down
- Indications
  - Repeat cesarean (elective; patient does not desire a trial of labor)
  - Dystocia or failure to progress in labor, breech or transverse lie
  - Concern for fetal well-being (i.e. fetal distress)
- *Vaginal birth after C-Section (VBAC):* Associated with a small but significant risk of uterine rupture, with poor outcome for mother and infant (higher risk with classical type)
  - *Candidates for VBAC:* One or two prior LTCSs, clinically adequate pelvis, no other uterine scars or previous rupture, physician available in case need of C-section
- *Indications for C-section:* Prolonged second stage, maternal heart disease, acute pulmonary edema, intrapartum infection, maternal aneurysm, prolapse of the cord, abnormal fetal heart rate, inadequate uterine contractions, abnormal positioning of fetal head, maternal exhaustion, or need to hasten delivery.
- *Indications for forceps delivery*
  - A fully dilated cervix, ruptured membranes, engaged fetal head, > +2 station, no cephalopelvic disproportion, empty bladder, and vertex presentation.

PRETERM LABOR

- Defined as gestational age (GA) <37 weeks with regular uterine contractions and:
    - 2 cm dilated/80% effaced cervix, progressing cervical changes or ruptured membranes.
- *Risks:* History of preterm labor, short cervix, bacterial vaginosis and multiple gestations
- *Prevention:*
    - Screen and treat high risk patients for bacterial vaginosis (Clindamycin 300 BID × 7 days, Metronidazole 500 mg BID × 7 days, Metronidazole 250 mg TID × 7 days).
    - Antenatal progesterone with history of prior preterm delivery or cervical length <15 mm.
    - Cervical cerclage addresses cervical structural causes of preterm labor.
- *Assessment of patients at risk of preterm labor:*
    - Check for rupture of membranes Ferning/Nitrizine), rule out infection (GBS carrier status, UTI), assess likelihood of premature delivery (cervical length by US).
- *Management:* Deliver at a facility with level III nursery
    - Dehydration causes antidiuretic hormone secretion, which mimics Oxytocin (both made in posterior pituitary). Rehydration can stop contractions.
    - Tocolytics used if <34 weeks to delay delivery to allow for steroids and GBS prophylaxis.

- ❖ *Contraindications:* Severe bleeding; abruptio placentae; fetal death, severe fetal anomaly; chorioamnionitis; severe gestational HTN; unstable maternal hemodynamics.
- Corticosteroids for lung maturation (Betamethasone 12 mg IM q d × 2 doses, if not available give Dexamethasone 6 mg IM q 12 hours × 4 doses). Do not repeat the steroids.
- *Prophylaxis of group B Strep:* Ampicillin 2 g IV then 1 g every 4 hours until delivery.

Give Tocolytics if under 34 Weeks

- *First line therapy:* Magnesium sulfate is calcium antagonist. Initial IV bolus of 4–6 g over 30 minutes, then a maintenance infusion of 1–3 g per hour.
  - Do not give in patients with myasthenia gravis or heart block. Be careful when administering in renal disease and recent heart attack.
  - *Side effects:* Depressed deep tendon reflexes (DTRs), pulmonary edema, nausea, flushing, headache and fatigue.
  - Mg level 4–7 mg/dL causes decreased uterine contractions. 8–12 mg/dL depresses deep tendon reflexes. >12 mg/dL respiratory/cardiac depression (treat with calcium gluconate).
- Indomethacin is a prostaglandin synthetase inhibitor. Add second line if Mg fails.

- Loading dose of 50-100 mg then 25-50 mg every 4 hours for 24 hours (maximum daily dose 200 mg). Peaks 1-2 hours after oral administration; following rectal administration levels peak slightly sooner.
- *High risk of side effects if given >48 hours:* Premature constriction of ductus arteriosus, pulmonary HTN, interventricular hemorrhage and oligohydramnios. *Recommended dosage:* 50-100 mg orally (initial dose), followed with 25-50 mg orally Q6 hours.
- Not past 30-32 weeks due to increased risk for side effects and necrotizing enterocolitis.
- *Beta-sympathomimetic:* Causes uterine smooth muscle relaxation by activation of beta2-receptors (also in blood vessels, bronchioles and liver). Delays delivery for 24-48 hours.
    - Terbutaline initial infusion 5-10 mg/minute, increase the dose when necessary to every 10-15 minutes to a maximum of 80 mg/minute, or Sq 0.25-mg q 20-30 minutes (4-6 doses).
    - *Relative contraindications:* Diabetes, cardiac disease, digitalis, hyperthyroid, HTN, and severe anemia. *Side effects:* Cardiac arrhythmias, pulmonary edema, and myocardial ischemia.
- *Calcium channel blockers* decrease uterine contractility
    - Nifedipine 20 mg orally initial, then 10-20 mg every 6-8 hours.
    - *Contraindications:* Hypotension, congestive heart failure, and aortic stenosis.

MAGNESIUM NOTE

- *S: Preterm labor (PTL) questions:* Ask about contractions, loss of fluid, vaginal bleeding, gross fetal movements, shortness of breath, cough and chest pain.
  - *Pre-eclampsia (PIH) questions:* Ask about headache, visual changes, RUQ pain, and edema.
  - *Mg toxicity questions:* Shortness of breath, weakness/drowsiness/lethargy/sleepiness.
- *O: VS (over 4 hours since last mag note):* T, BP, P, RR, O2 Sat, urine output (UOP)/hour (worrisome if <30). In patients with pre-eclampsia, note BP ranges.
- *PE:* General: awake (?); alert (?); distress (?)
- *Pulm:* Clear to auscultation bilaterally (CTAB) (?)
- *CV:* Rate/rhythm (?); murmurs/rubs/gallops (m/r/g) (?)
- *Abd:* RUQ tenderness (?)
- *Ext:* Edema/calf tenderness (?); DTRs (increases in PIH, decreased Mg) (?); clonus (?)
- *FHT:* Baseline, variability, reactivity (?); accelerations/decelerations (?); category of FHT (?)
- *Tocometer (external/internal):* Frequency of contractions, intrauterine pressure in Montevideo units (MvUs)
- *Labs:* (only if new labs)
- *A/P:* ____yo G__P__ with PIH at ____weeks, _____ presentation. No s/s of Mg toxicity.
  - Continue Mg. Recheck patient again in __ hours.
  - Preterm labor (PTL)?—Contractions (ctx)? Cervix: changed/unchanged.
  - For PIH—stable (Y/N). BP? Stable: Hydralazine/Labetalol for BP > 160/110.
  - Follow labs (HELLP labs, etc.)

MANAGEMENT OF PREMATURES RUPTURE OF MEMBRANES

- *For all PROM patients:* Evaluate patient for chorioamnionitis (common cause):
    - Fever > 38°C, leukocytosis, maternal/fetal tachycardia, uterine tenderness, malodorous vaginal discharge.
    - Obtain amniotic fluid Gram stain and culture.
    - If chorioamnionitis is diagnosed, deliver despite gestational age, and give antibiotics (Ampicillin, Gentamicin).

Premature Rupture of Membranes

90% go into labor within 24 hours of rupture, and are allowed to progress. If labor is not spontaneous, it should be induced or consider C-section.

Preterm Premature Rupture of Membranes

- Balance the risks of premature birth against the risk of infection.
    - Gram stain and culture of amniotic fluid to assess for chorioamnionitis
    - *Antibiotics:*
        - Ampicillin 2 g IV every 6 hours × 48 hours then 250 mg PO every 8 hours × 5 days or
        - Erythromycin 250 mg IV every 6 hours × 48 hours then 333 mg PO every 8 hours × 5 days
    - Amniotic fluid assessment of lecithin—sphingomyelin ratio for lung maturity.

- Perform ultrasound to assess gestational age, position of baby and AFI.
- If <34 weeks, give steroids to decrease incidence of respiratory distress syndrome (RDS).

LABOR DYSTOCIA

- Slow progression of labor, caused by:
  - *Abnormalities of the expulsive forces:* Uterine forces too weak or uncoordinated, or inadequate voluntary muscle effort during second stage of labor (powers)
  - Abnormal fetal presentation, position, or development (passenger issues)
  - Abnormalities of the maternal bony pelvis or birth canal (passage issues)
- Prolonged latent phase >20 hours in nulliparous or >14 hours multiparous
  - Treat with maternal rest or with Oxytocin
- Active phase abnormalities—may be due to cephalopelvic disproportion (CPD), excessive sedation, conduction analgesia and fetal malposition [persistent occiput posterior (OP) position]
  - Protraction disorders—slower than average cervical dilation or fetal descent
    - Dilation <1.2 cm/h or descent <1 cm/h in nulliparous
    - Dilation <1.5 cm/h or descent <2 cm/h in multiparous

- Arrest disorders—complete cessation of dilation or descent for
  - Longer than 4 hours for nulliparous with epidural
  - Over 3 hours for nulliparous without epidural or multiparous with epidural
  - More than 2 hours for nulliparous without epidural
- *Management:*
  - If cephalopelvic dysproportion (CPD), deliver by C-section.
  - Without CPD, augment labor with Oxytocin. Begin at 0.5–2 mIU/min, increase by 1–2 mIU every 15–30 minutes until adequate contraction pattern or 8–10 mIU/min. Observe for one hour and if still inadequate, increase to 20 mIU/min. MAX 32 mIU/min (weigh risks).

ABNORMAL THIRD STAGE OF LABOR

- Abnormal placentation is the abnormal implantation of the placenta in the uterus
  - *Risk factors:* Placenta previa, previous C-section, previous dilation and curettage (D&C), grand multiparity.
  - Often these disorders result in postpartum hemorrhage and require hysterectomy.
  - Types
    - *Placenta accreta:* The placental villi attach directly to the myometrium rather than to the decidua basalis.

- *Placenta increta:* The placental villi invade the myometrium.
- *Placenta percreta:* The placental villi penetrate through the myometrium.
- *Uterine inversion:*
  - Often results from too much traction while delivering the placenta, or as a result of abnormal placental implantation. Morbidity results from shock and sepsis.
  - *Management:* Remove the placenta. Replace the inverted uterus by pushing upward on the fundus toward the vagina and when it is fully replaced give Oxytocin.
- Macrosomia is birth weight >4,500 g.
  - *Risk factors:* Diabetes, obesity, previous history, postdates pregnancy, multiparity and advanced maternal age.
  - *Macrosomic infants are at risk for:* Birth trauma, jaundice, hypoglycemia, low Apgar scores and childhood tumors.
  - Mothers are at risk for increased birth trauma and postpartum hemorrhage.

POSTPARTUM HEMORRHAGE

- Immediate postpartum hemorrhage (>500 mL in vaginal delivery, >1 L for C-section)
  - *During first 24 hours:* "Early" postpartum hemorrhage.
  - *From 24 hours to 6 weeks after delivery:* "Late" postpartum hemorrhage.

Abnormal Labor

- Most common cause is uterine atony. Uterus cannot contract enough to compress the blood vessels and prevent bleeding.
  Other causes: Coagulation defects, ruptured uterus, uterine inversion, retained placental tissue or genital tract trauma.
- *Risk factors:* Previous hemorrhage with delivery, coagulopathy, vaginal birth after C-section, macrosomia, and high parity.
- *Management:*
  - Bimanually massage the uterus, which controls most cases of atony.
  - Give Oxytocin (20 units in 1 L of lactated Ringer's) or Methergine 0.2 IM, or Hemabate 0.25 IM, or Cytotec (misoprostol) 1000 mcg rectally.
  - Look at the blood, if not clotting—give factors, FFP, platelets, and factor VIIa.
  - Perform manual exploration of the uterus to ensure all placental parts are delivered.
  - Inspect the cervix and vagina to rule out trauma/lacerations, and ensure the uterus is intact and not inverted.
  - Blood loss 1-1.5 L or more is massive hemorrhage. Place Foley and monitor urine output. Take blood for typing and crossmatching and begin fluid or blood replacement. Support blood pressure with vasopressors. Perform uterine packing.
  - *Last resort:* Exploratory laparotomy, hysterectomy, embolization of pelvic vessels or uterine artery/hypogastric artery ligation.

SHOULDER DYSTOCIA

Shoulder dystocia: The fetal shoulder is impacted behind the pubic symphysis after the head delivers.

- *Risk factors:* Macrosomia, gestational diabetes, maternal obesity, post-term delivery, prolonged stage 2 of labor.
- *Complications:* Fetal humeral/clavicular fracture, brachial plexus nerve injuries, hypoxia/death.
- Several maneuvers can be done to displace the shoulder impaction:
  - Suprapubic pressure on maternal abdomen
  - *McRoberts maneuver:* Maternal thighs are sharply flexed against maternal abdomen. This decreases the angle between the sacrum and spine and may dislodge fetal shoulder.
  - *Woods corkscrew maneuver:* Pressure is applied against scapula of posterior shoulder to rotate the posterior shoulder and "unscrew" the anterior shoulder.
  - *Posterior shoulder delivery:* Hand is inserted into vagina and posterior arm is pulled across chest, delivering posterior shoulder and displacing anterior shoulder from behind pubic symphysis
  - Break clavicle or cut through symphysis.
  - *Zavanelli maneuver:* If the above measures do not work, the fetal head can be returned to the uterus. At this point, a C-section would be performed.

BREECH

- In breech presentations, the presenting fetal part is the buttocks. Those found early in pregnancy will often spontaneously convert to vertex as term approaches.
- *Risk factors:* Low birth weight (20–30% of breeches), congenital anomalies, uterine anomalies, multiple gestation, placenta previa.
- *Diagnosis can be made by:* Leopold maneuvers and ultrasound.
- Types of breech position:
  - *Frank breech (65%):* Feet are in front of the head or face
  - *Complete breech (25%):* The thighs lay on the abdomen and the legs are flexed as well so that the feet are by the buttocks.
  - *Incomplete (footling) breech (10%):* One or both of the hips are not flexed so that a foot lies below.
- Normally, C-section is the form of delivery. An experienced provider can perform external cephalic version to maneuver the infant to a vertex position. Can be done only if breech is diagnosed before onset of labor and the GA >37 weeks. The success rate is 75%, and the risks are placental abruption or cord compression.
- *Trial of breech vaginal delivery:* This is the attempt at a vaginal delivery. It can be done only in a frank breech, GA >36 weeks, fetal weight 2,500–3,800 g, fetal head flexed, and favorable pelvis. Risks are greater for birth trauma (especially brachial plexus injuries) and prolapsed cord that entraps the head.

BIBLIOGRAPHY

ACOG Committee on Obstetric Practice. ACOG Committee Opinion No. 340. Mode of term singleton breech delivery. Obstet Gynecol. 2006;108:235.

ACOG committee opinion no. 561: Nonmedically indicated early-term deliveries. Obstet Gynecol. 2013;121:911.

American College of Obstetricians and Gynecologists, Committee on Practice Bulletins—Obstetrics. ACOG practice bulletin no. 127: Management of preterm labor. Obstet Gynecol. 2012;119:1308.

American College of Obstetricians and Gynecologists. ACOG Committee opinion #529. Placenta accreta. Obstet Gynecol. 2012;120:207.

American College of Obstetricians and Gynecologists. ACOG Practice Bulletin: Clinical Management Guidelines for postpartum hemorrhage. Obstet Gynecol. 2006;76(108):1039.

American College of Obstetricians and Gynecologists. Management of preterm labor. ACOG Practice Bulletin. 43, 2003.

Baskett TF. Acute uterine inversion: a review of 40 cases. J Obstet Gynaecol Can. 2002;24:953.

Borna S, Sahabi N. Progesterone for maintenance tocolytic therapy after threatened preterm labour: a randomised controlled trial. Aust N Z J Obstet Gynaecol. 2008;48:58.

Cheng YW, Shaffer BL, Bryant AS, Caughey AB. Length of the first stage of labor and associated perinatal outcomes in nulliparous women. Obstet Gynecol. 2010;116:1127.

Costley PL, East CE. Oxytocin augmentation of labour in women with epidural analgesia for reducing operative deliveries. Cochrane Database Syst Rev. 2013;7.

Dennedy MC, Dunne F. Macrosomia: defining the problem worldwide. Lancet. 2013;381:435.

Ellestad SC, Swamy GK, Sinclair T, et al. Preterm premature rupture of membrane management—inpatient versus outpatient: a retrospective review. Am J Perinatol. 2008;25:69.

Fiori O, Deux JF, Kambale JC, et al. Impact of pelvic arterial embolization for intractable postpartum hemorrhage on fertility. Am J Obstet Gynecol. 2009;200:384.e1.

Goldenberg RL. Arrested preterm labor: do the data support home or hospital care? Obstet Gynecol. 2005;106:3.

Haas DM, Imperiale TF, Kirkpatrick PR, et al. Tocolytic therapy: a meta-analysis and decision analysis. Obstet Gynecol. 2009;113:585.

Han S, Crowther CA, Moore V. Magnesium maintenance therapy for preventing preterm birth after threatened preterm labour. Cochrane Database Syst Rev. 2013.

Hannah ME, Hannah WJ, Hewson SA, et al. Planned caesarean section versus planned vaginal birth for breech presentation at term: a randomised multicentre trial. Term Breech Trial Collaborative Group. Lancet. 2000;356:1375.

Hoffman MK, Bailit JL, Branch DW, et al. A comparison of obstetric maneuvers for the acute management of shoulder dystocia. Obstet Gynecol. 2011;117:1272.

Jansen AJ, van Rhenen DJ, Steegers EA, Duvekot JJ. Postpartum hemorrhage and transfusion of blood and blood components. Obstet Gynecol Surv. 2005;60:663.

National Institutes of Health Consensus Development Conference Statement. NIH Consensus Development Conference: Vaginal Birth After Cesarean: New Insights, March 8–10, 2010.

Osmundson SS, Garabedian MJ, Lyell DJ. Risk factors for classical hysterotomy by gestational age. Obstet Gynecol. 2013;122:845.

Oyelese Y, Smulian JC. Placenta previa, placenta accreta, and vasa previa. Obstet Gynecol. 2006;107:927.

Paris AE, Greenberg JA, Ecker JL, McElrath TF. Is an episiotomy necessary with a shoulder dystocia? Am J Obstet Gynecol. 2011;205:217.e1.

Parry S, Strauss JF 3rd. Premature rupture of the fetal membranes. N Engl J Med. 1998;338:663.

Passos F, Cardoso K, Coelho AM, et al. Antibiotic prophylaxis in premature rupture of membranes at term: a randomized controlled trial. Obstet Gynecol. 2012;120:1045.

Poggi SH, Allen RH, Patel CR, et al. Randomized trial of McRoberts versus lithotomy positioning to decrease the force that is applied to the fetus during delivery. Am J Obstet Gynecol. 2004;191:874.

Rouse DJ, Owen J, Savage KG, Hauth JC. Active phase labor arrest: revisiting the 2-hour minimum. Obstet Gynecol. 2001;98:550.

Toivonen E, Palomäki O, Huhtala H, Uotila J. Selective vaginal breech delivery at term—still an option. Acta Obstet Gynecol Scand 2012;91:1177.

University Hospitals Case Medical Center, MacDonald Women's Hospital. Resident's Manual; 2007.

Vogel JP, West HM, Dowswell T. Titrated oral misoprostol for augmenting labour to improve maternal and neonatal outcomes. Cochrane Database Syst Rev. 2013; 9.

Wei SQ, Luo ZC, Qi HP, et al. High-dose vs low-dose oxytocin for labor augmentation: a systematic review. Am J Obstet Gynecol. 2010;203:296.

Zhang J, Troendle J, Mikolajczyk R, et al. The natural history of the normal first stage of labor. Obstet Gynecol. 2010;115:705.

5
Postpartum

CHAPTER OUTLINES

- Immediate Postdelivery Tasks
- Routine Postpartum Care
- Discharge Planning
- Postpartum Maternal Changes
- Breastfeeding
- Postpartum Infections
- Postpartum Psychiatric Complications

IMMEDIATE POSTDELIVERY TASKS

- Clear the infant's nasopharynx with a bulb syringe to minimize aspiration.
- Clamp and cut the cord (or allow family member to cut) between the two clamps.
- Hand the baby to the pediatrician/nurse for examination/resuscitation.
- Sample of cord blood from the placental side is collected and sent to the lab.
- *Deliver the placenta:* Give Oxytocin, gentle cord traction, perform fundal massage.
- Repair lacerations to the perineum and anus caused by stretching and thinning.

- *Prevention with episiotomy:* Incision placed prior to delivery. Two types—midline (most common) and mediolateral (oblique at 5 o'clock). Indications—risk of rupture, shoulder dystocia, breech or assisted delivery.
- *First degree:* Involves the Fourchette, perineal skin, and vaginal mucosa, but not the underlying fascia and muscle. Repair with absorbable sutures like 3-0 vicryl.
- *Second degree:* First degree plus the fascia and muscle of the perineal body but not the anal sphincter. Repair in layers to bring the perineal body together (3-0).
- *Third degree:* Second degree plus involvement of the anal sphincter. Repair anal sphincter with interrupted sutures (2-0 vicryl) and repair vagina in layers with 3-0.
- *Fourth degree:* Extends through the rectal mucosa to expose the lumen of the rectum. Repair the same as third degree plus repair of rectal mucosa (4-0 vicryl).
- *Hemostasis:* Uses myometrial contraction to cause vasoconstriction.
  - Oxytocin, fundal massage to increase myometrial contractions and reduce maternal blood loss. Gentle cord traction promotes placental separation.

ROUTINE POSTPARTUM CARE

First Hour

- Check maternal BP and HR at least every 15 minutes. Monitor the amount of vaginal bleeding. Fundal massage through the abdominal wall.

First Several Hours

- Early ambulation leads to less bladder complications, decreased constipation, reduced risk of DVT and PE. Mom can eat as soon as 2 hours postdelivery.
- New mom should void within 4 hours of delivery. If not an indwelling catheter may be necessary, with prophylactic antibiotic after catheter removal.
- *For a repaired laceration:* Apply an ice pack to reduce edema and pain until 24 hours postpartum, then apply moist heat (warm sitz baths) to decrease discomfort.

The First Few Days

- Lack of bowel movement may be due to bowel cleanse prior to delivery. Encourage early ambulation and eating.
- If fourth degree laceration fecal incontinence may be due to injury to the pelvic floor.
- Pain can be due to labor after pains, laceration repair, breast engorgement, or postspinal puncture headache. Treat with codeine and acetaminophen.
- Rh-negative mom with Rh-positive baby receives immunoglobin within 72 hours of delivery.
- If no history of rubella immunity, vaccinate mom prior to discharge, consider Tdap booster.
- Iron supplementation for a minimum of 3 months postpartum.

DISCHARGE PLANNING

- Prior to discharge, make follow-up appointments for mom and baby.
  - Newborn should receive the initial HBV vaccine and all screening tests (like PKU).
- After hospital discharge, the patient should return if she experiences fever, excessive vaginal bleeding, lower extremity pain and/or swelling, shortness of breath and chest pain.

Family Planning and Contraception

- Contraception should be started before the first menses as ovulation can restart prior to resumption of menses, unless a subsequent pregnancy is desired.
- The lactational amenorrhea method is 98% effective for up to 6 months if the mother is not menstruating and if the baby is nursing 2–3 times nightly and at least every 4 hours during the day without other supplementation.
- Combined oral contraceptive hormones reduce the amount of breast milk, although very small quantities of the hormones are excreted in the milk.
- Progestin only oral contraceptive pills are virtually 100% effective without substantially reducing the amount of breast milk.
- May resume coitus after 6 weeks with a vaginal lubricant for comfort.
  - Premature intercourse can cause pain due to laceration/scar healing and due to continued uterine

involution. There is also a risk of hemorrhage and infection.

POSTPARTUM MATERNAL CHANGES

- *Uterus:* Fundus begins to contract from delivery and returns to normal size in 2 weeks.
- *Endometrium:* Superficial layer sloughs off as red *lochia rubra* for 3 days postpartum. *Lochia serosa* is paler, from days 4–10 and *lochia alba* (white to yellow) from day 11 on until the basal layer becomes the new endometrial layer.
- *Placental site:* Uterine side contains many thrombosed vessels that decrease in size from palm sized to 4 cm diameter by 2 weeks postpartum.
- New, smaller vessels due to hyaline changes replace uterine blood vessels.
- *Cervix:* External os is narrowed at one week.
- *Lower uterine segment:* Contracts and retracts to normal size within 3 weeks.
- Vaginal outlet gradually diminishes in size, but rarely returns to its nulliparous state.
- Vaginal rugae reappear by week 3 but after repeated childbirth may not return.
- *Abdominal wall:* It recovers from distention within 2 months.
- *Urinary tract:* Bladder has increased capacity and low pressure. Dilated ureters and renal pelvices lead to increased UTI risk (these constrict by 8 weeks postpartum).
- *Fluid diuresis:* Total body fluid returns to nonpregnant range in 1 week.

- *Leukocytosis* during and after labor up to 30,000/µL, with a relative lymphopenia.
- *Cardiac output* remains elevated for ≥ 48 hours postpartum.
- *Weight changes* approach normal by 6 months.

BREASTFEEDING

- Contraindications:
    - *Infection:* Cytomegalovirus (CMV), chronic hepatitis B (HBV), HIV infection, breast lesions from active herpes simplex virus.
    - *Medications:* Bromocriptine, Cyclophosphamide, Cyclosporine, Doxorubicin, Ergotamine, Lithium, Methotrexate.
    - *Meds with unknown effects:* Psychotropic drugs, antianxiety medications, antidepressants, Chloramphenicol, Metoclopramide, Metronidazole, Tinidazole.
    - *Drug abuse:* Amphetamines, cocaine, heroin, marijuana, nicotine, Phencyclidine.
    - *Radiotherapy:* Gallium, indium, iodine, radioactive sodium, technetium.
- Benefits:
    - Nursing accelerates uterine involution and lactating mothers use 500 extra calories daily.
    - Colostrum and breast milk contain secretory IgA, memory T cells, IL-6, growth factor.
    - Infants easily absorb breast milk, and it contains all essential and nonessential amino acids.

- Stages of breast milk:
  - Colostrum can be expressed from the nipple by the second postpartum day and is secreted by the breasts for 5 days postpartum.
  - This matures to milk by 4 weeks postpartum. Subsequent lactation is controlled by prolactin and repetitive stimulus of nursing.

POSTPARTUM INFECTIONS

- *Possible signs:* Fever > 100.4°F (38°C), soft, tender uterus, foul-smelling lochia, leukocytosis (WBC > 10,000/µL), malaise.
- *Management:* Identify source and cause of infection, treat with antibiotics.
- *Endometritis:*
  - Uterine infection involving the decidua, myometrium and parametrial tissue. Typically develops postpartum day 2–3. Treat with IV antibiotics (Gentamicin and Clindamycin) until patient is afebrile for 24–48 hours.
- *C-section skin infection:*
  - Wound erythema, tenderness, fever on postoperative day 4 or 5 suggests wound infection. Obtain Gram stain and cultures from wound, then drain, irrigate and debride the wound. Start antibiotics if extensive infection is suspected.
- *Laceration or episiotomy infection:*
  - Pain at the site, scar disruption, or a necrotic membrane over the wound signals possible infection.

Rule out a rectovaginal fistula with both rectal and vaginal exams. Open, clean, and debride the wound to promote healing. Sitz baths for cleaning open areas and reconsider closing after granulation tissue has appeared.
- *Mastitis:*
  - Epidemic mastitis is caused by infant with nasal colonization of *Staphylococcus aureus*. Mother presents with fever and breast tenderness on postpartum day 2-4. Treat with Penicillin.
  - Endemic mastitis—weeks or months after delivery. Mother presents with fever, systemic illness, and breast tenderness. Treat with Penicillin or Dicloxacillin. Continue breastfeeding.

POSTPARTUM PSYCHIATRIC COMPLICATIONS

- *Postpartum blues*
  - A mild depression that begins 3-6 days after delivery and lasts up to 10 days.
  - Support the patient—acknowledge her feelings and reassure.
  - Monitor for symptoms of postpartum depression or psychosis.
- *Postpartum depression*
  - Same criteria and symptoms as minor and major depression, but it also begin within 3-6 months after childbirth. Symptoms will gradually improve over 6 months with antidepressants, anxiolytics and possibly electroconvulsive therapy.

- Comanage patient with a psychiatrist for psychotherapy to focus on any maternal fears or concerns.
- *Postpartum psychosis*
  - Mothers have an inability to discern reality from fantasy (may have periods of lucidity).
  - *Peak onset:* 10 to 14 days postpartum, but may occur months later. Duration is variable and depends on underlying mental illness, but often lasts 6 months.
  - Risk factors include a personal or family history of psychiatric illness, mothers of younger age, primiparity.
  - Treat with psychiatric care, pharmacotherapy and hospitalization for most patients.

BIBLIOGRAPHY

American Academy of Pediatrics, American College of Obstetricians and Gynecologists. Guidelines for Perinatal Care, 7th edn 2012.

Bloch M, Rotenberg N, Koren D, Klein E. Risk factors associated with the development of postpartum mood disorders. J Affect Disord. 2005;88:9.

Breastfeeding in the Hospital: The Postpartum Period. In: Breastfeeding Handbook for Physicians, AAP/ACOG. 2006.

Brockington I. Postpartum psychiatric disorders. Lancet. 2004;363:303.

Brown S, Lumley J. Maternal health after childbirth: results of an Australian population based survey. Br J Obstet Gynaecol. 1998;105:156.

Chiong Tan P, Jin Norazilah M, Zawiah Omar S. Hospital discharge on the first compared with the second day after a planned cesarean delivery: a randomized controlled trial. Obstet Gynecol. 2012;120:1273.

Committee on Health Care for Underserved Women, American College of Obstetricians and Gynecologists. ACOG Committee Opinion No.

361: Breastfeeding: maternal and infant aspects. Obstet Gynecol. 2007;109:479.

Committee on Obstetric Practice, American College of Obstetricians and Gynecologists. Committee Opinion No. 543: Timing of umbilical cord clamping after birth. Obstet Gynecol. 2012;120:1522.

Da Costa D, Larouche J, Dritsa M, Brender W. Psychosocial correlates of prepartum and postpartum depressed mood. J Affect Disord. 2000;59:31.

Groen RS, Bae JY, Lim KJ. Fear of the unknown: ionizing radiation exposure during pregnancy. Am J Obstet Gynecol. 2012;206:456.

Landy HJ, Laughon SK, Bailit JL, et al. Characteristics associated with severe perineal and cervical lacerations during vaginal delivery. Obstet Gynecol. 2011;117:627.

Minig L, Trimble EL, Sarsotti C, et al. Building the evidence base for postoperative and postpartum advice. Obstet Gynecol. 2009;114:892.

Owen J, Andrews WW. Wound complications after cesarean sections. Clin Obstet Gynecol. 1994;37:842.

Resnik R. The Puerperium. In: Creasy RK, Resnik R (Eds). Maternal Fetal-Medicine, Principles and Practice, Saunders WB. Philadelphia, 2004. p. 165.

Sachs HC. Committee on Drugs. The transfer of drugs and therapeutics into human breast milk: an update on selected topics. Pediatrics. 2013;132:e796.

Sarsam SE, Elliott JP, Lam GK. Management of wound complications from cesarean delivery. Obstet Gynecol Surv. 2005;60:462.

Sheldon WR, Durocher J, Winikoff B, et al. How effective are the components of active management of the third stage of labor? BMC Pregnancy Childbirth. 2013;13:46.

Signorello LB, Harlow BL, Chekos AK, Repke JT. Postpartum sexual functioning and its relationship to perineal trauma: a retrospective cohort study of primiparous women. Am J Obstet Gynecol. 2001;184:881.

Spencer JP. Management of mastitis in breastfeeding women. Am Fam Physician. 2008;78:727.

Thompson JF, Roberts CL, Currie M, Ellwood DA. Prevalence and persistence of health problems after childbirth: associations with parity and method of birth. Birth. 2002;29:83.

6

Gynecology Consult

CHAPTER OUTLINES

- Gynecologic Clinic Note
- Complete Gynecologic History
- Procedure and Postoperative Notes
- Postoperative Concerns in Gynecology
- Uterine Bleeding
- Dysfunctional Uterine Bleeding
- Menopause
- Pre- and Postmenopausal Bleeding
- Pelvic Pain (Acute and Chronic)
- Pelvic Inflammatory Disease
- Toxic Shock Syndrome
- Incontinence and Pelvic Organ Prolapse
- Gestational Trophoblastic Disease
- Ovarian Cyst Management
- Cancer Screening Don'ts
- Cervical Dysplasia Classification
- Gynecologic Cancer
- Cervical Cancer FIGO Staging
- Endometrial Cancer FIGO Staging
- Ovarian Cancer FIGO Staging
- Vaginal and Vulvar Cancer FIGO Staging

GYNECOLOGIC CLINIC NOTE

- *HPI:* Age GP with LMP date presents for __. Expand on any issues regarding onset, duration, frequency, etc.
- *OB/GYN Hx*
- *Menstrual history*
- *Sexual history to include h/o STDs, PID:* List which, date(s), treatment(s).

Gynecology Consult

- *Pap hx:* Last Pap and result, h/o any abnormal Pap smears and if so what treatment was offered.
- *MMG hx:* Last mammogram date and result, any abnormal and what treatments.
- *DEXA scan hx:* Any scans with date and result.
- *Gyn surg hx:* Any gyn surgeries and for what indication (i.e. dx lap for pelvic pain, TAH for fibroids, Burch for SUI, D&C for menorrhagia, etc.).
- Urinary or fecal incontinence.
- PMH, PSH, SH, Meds, Allergies, ROS.
- *FH:* Usual medical problems + Breast Ca, Colon Ca, Gyn Ca – if yes, note family member on maternal/paternal side, and age/decade of diagnosis if known.
- Vitals/Exam as indicated.
- *Assessment:* Age, G, P with diagnoses.
- *Plan:* Include when to return for follow-up.

COMPLETE GYNECOLOGIC HISTORY

- *Menstrual history:* Age at menarche, the duration of menstrual flow (normal is 3–7 days), the interval of the cycle (normal is 28–35 days), and the amount of flow.
- *Last menstrual period (LMP):* The date of the first day of bleeding of the last period and describe any abnormality of her menses.
- *Postmenopausal:* Date of last menses and presence of menopausal symptoms.
- *Pelvic infections:* PID, STDs (Gonorrhea, Chlamydia, Syphilis, Herpes, Hepatitis, HPV, HIV, etc.). Record date of

infection and if infection was/is being treated. Also history of other infections, such as yeast, trichomoniasis, bacterial vaginosis, etc.
- *Genital neoplasm:* Any tumors or growths on the external or internal genitalia.
- *Endometriosis:* History of diagnosis, treatment modalities.
- *Pap history:* Last Pap smear, history of abnormal Pap smears, treatments to the cervix (LEEP, Cones, Cryo, etc.).
- *Mammogram history:* Last mammogram, history of abnormal scans, ultrasounds, biopsies, FNAs, etc.
- *Fertility:* And history of difficulty with conception, assisted reproduction, etc.
- *Sexual history:* Is patient sexually active, what is sexual orientation, how may life partners, how many current partners, how many partners in last 12 months, age at first intercourse, satisfaction with sex-life, orgasmic complaints, history of rape or sexual abuse, or physical or emotional abuse, methods of contraception and STD prevention.

PROCEDURE AND POSTOPERATIVE NOTES

- Procedure note
  - Preoperative Dx (e.g. Endometrial cancer)
  - Postoperative Dx (same)
  - Procedure (total abdominal hysterectomy, bilateral salpingo-oophorectomy, pelvic and para-aortic lymphadenectomy)
  - Attending: ___ Assistant (Resident)
  - Anesthesia: General endotracheal anesthesia

- EBL: [100 cc] IVF: [2500 cc LR] UOP: [150 cc]
- Specimens (uterus, tubes, ovaries, lymph nodes)
- Drains (none, etc.); Complications: none
- Disposition: Patient sent to recovery in stable condition
- Postoperative note
  - *Subjective:* Record patient complaints and ROS including pain levels.
  - *Objective:* Vitals—record current temp/maximum temp, as well as other vitals.
  - *Urine output:* Urine output should be at least 30 cc/hr.
  - *Wound:* Note excessive drainage or frank bleeding and presence and functionality of drains.
  - *Drain output:* Note volume and quality of drain output (serosanguinous, etc.)
  - *Labs:* Any labs (e.g. H/H) drawn after surgery or that are pending.
  - *Assessment/Plan:* [POD#0 s/p TAH/BSO/PPLND secondary to _____ condition. Path pending. Pt. stable, adequate pain relief on __. UOP adequate. H/H trend?]
  - *Plan for daily progress note:* [Add planned treatments or procedures for the day, i.e. remove Foley, ambulate, advance diet, iron, IVF, antiemetics, HRT, D/C, labs, etc.]

POSTOPERATIVE CONCERNS IN GYNECOLOGY

- Complications include hemorrhage, infection, DVT and damage to nearby organs.

- Abdominal surgery
  - Staples and skin sutures are generally removed between 3 and 10 days postoperative.
  - Steri-strips can be removed one week after surgery.
  - Bandages can be removed 24–48 hours after the procedure.
  - Incisions should be gently cleaned with running water. No soap needed, and no direct scrubbing to avoid scar disruption.
- Vaginal surgery
  - Vaginal stitches are absorbable and will not need to be removed.
  - Light vaginal bleeding or discharge is normal for up to a month.
- *Pain* is typically controlled with anti-inflammatory medications
  - For severe pain that may be experienced with hysterectomy or major surgeries, pain pumps may be placed during surgery, and limited course of narcotics may be needed.
- Lifting is limited to under 15 lbs for 6 weeks.
- Pelvic rest (no intercourse or tampons) for 6 weeks.
- Any drains placed will be managed by the surgeon but make sure to note the type, location, amount and color of drainage.

UTERINE BLEEDING

- *Polymenorrhea:* Menses with regular intervals that are under 18 days.

- *Menorrhagia:* Menses over 7 days in duration, or excess blood loss (>80 mL) at normal intervals. Causes include leiomyoma, adenomyosis, cervical cancer, coagulopathy, endometrial hyperplasia, endometrial cancer or polyps.
- *Hypermenorrhea:* Menses over 7 days in duration, or excess blood loss (>80 mL) at regular but not always normal intervals.
- *Hypomenorrhea:* Decreased menstrual flow.
- *Oligomenorrhea:* Menses with more than 35 day intervals between cycles.
- *Metrorrhagia:* Bleeding at irregular intervals; intermenstrual bleeding. Causes include polyps, increased estrogen levels, neoplasia or contraceptive complications.
- *Menometrorrhagia:* Combination of both menorrhagia and metrorrhagia; menses too long in duration or excessive blood loss and irregular bleeding intervals.
- *Kleine regnung:* Bleeding for 1-2 days during ovulation (scant).
- *Dysmenorrhea:* Painful menstrual flow. Treat with NSAIDs and contraceptives.
- *Intermenstrual bleeding:* Bleeding between regular intervals.
- *Amenorrhea:* Absence of menses.

DYSFUNCTIONAL UTERINE BLEEDING

- Abnormal uterine bleeding (AUB) unrelated to anatomic lesions; usually caused by hormonal dysfunction. It is a diagnosis made by exclusion after workup for anatomic causes of AUB.

- DUB is classified as either anovulatory or ovulatory:
  - Anovulation results in constant endometrial proliferation without progesterone-mediated maturation and shedding. The "overgrown" endometrium continually and irregularly sheds. Causes include: Polycystic ovaries, obesity, or unopposed estrogen.
    - *Ovulatory DUB:* Inadequate progesterone secretion by corpus luteum causes a luteal-phase defect and often presents with polymenorrhea or metrorrhagia.
    - *Workup:* Thorough menstrual and reproductive history, signs of systemic disease (thyroid, liver, kidney), extreme exercise, weight changes, presence or absence of ovulation (regularity, premenstrual body changes).
    - Treat with high-dose oral contraceptives or Medroxyprogesterone acetate ≥10 days
  - *Anovulatory:* Oral contraceptives mimic the normal menstrual cycle changes to allow for endometrial maturation and sloughing.
  - *Ovulatory:* NSAIDs are useful.
    - If medical treatment fails perform D&C, endometrial ablation or hysterectomy.
- Considerations in bleeding:
  - *Postcoital bleeding in pregnant woman:* Consider placenta previa.
  - *Postcoital bleeding in nonpregnant woman:* Consider cervical cancer.

MENOPAUSE

- Record date of cessation of menses and any menopausal symptoms.
- *Hot flashes:* Most frequently occurring symptom of sudden, episodic skin flushing and perspiration. Last 3-4 minutes, once a day up to 3 episodes per hour.
- *Lower urinary tract atrophy:* Atrophy of urethra and periurethra, loss of pelvic tone, prolapse of urethrovesicular junction. Symptoms of dysuria, urgency, frequency, suprapubic discomfort, frequent stress and urge incontinence.
- *Genital changes:* Shortening of vaginal canal, loss of vaginal folds, epithelial thinning and friability, bacterial vaginosis common. Leads to atrophic vaginitis, dyspareunia or vaginal bleeding.
- *Osteoporosis:* Associated with decreased bone mass, increased susceptibility to fractures. Estrogen supplementation decreases fracture risk by 50%.
- *Dyspareunia:* New or longstanding? Introital or with penetration?
- *Pelvic pain:* Ask about duration, location, quality, associated symptoms, what makes better or worse, etc.
- Women with vaginal atrophy or moderate to severe vasomotor symptoms without breast cancer or cardiovascular disease can be given short course of hormonal replacement therapy (HRT)
    - If the patient still has a uterus—add progestin
    - For vaginal atrophy—use vaginal estrogen only if lubricants or moisturizers are ineffective.

PRE- AND POSTMENOPAUSAL BLEEDING

- Premenopausal vaginal bleeding:
    - Consider PCOS as a likely cause.
    - If hCG positive and painful is likely a ruptured ectopic pregnancy—need urgent ultrasound.
    - Very high beta-hCG without fetal heartbeat is likely gestational trophoblastic neoplasia.
    - Beta-hCG positive +/- pain could be threatened/inevitable/incomplete abortion or ectopic.
- Look for products of conception in vagina (abortion), perform serial beta-hCG levels.
- Normal pregnancies have 2/3 rise in beta-hCG in 48 hours, in ectopic beta-hCG raise slower.
- *Beta-hCG negative:* Check PT/PTT, CT/US for pelvic mass, androgen levels and LH/FSH ratio for PCOS.
- *Postmenopausal vaginal bleeding:* Consider endometrial cancer as a likely cause. This bleeding begins more than 1 year after menopause.
- Differential diagnoses:
    - Endometrial hyperplasia
    - Cancer—cervical or vulvar
    - Estrogen-secreting tumor
    - Vaginal atrophy (most common)
- Workup:
    - Perform pelvic ultrasound
    - Endometrial biopsy and endocervical curettage because of the danger of cancer
    - Pap smear and colposcopy for cervical neoplasia

- *Imaging:* Consider ultrasound (transabdominal and transvaginal), hysteroscopy and/or computed tomography (CT) to assess spread of cervical and/or endometrial cancer.

PELVIC PAIN (ACUTE AND CHRONIC)

- **Chronic pelvic pain** is ≥6 months of pain, with incomplete relief by medical measures and altered activities like missed work, depression, sexual dysfunction.
  - *Causes:* Adnexal lesions, endometriosis, Müllerian anomalies, ovulatory pain, dysmenorrhea. Also consider urologic, GI, and MSK causes, neoplasia, leiomyoma, adhesions, adenomyosis, pelvic inflammatory disease (PID) and other infections.
  - Work-up in addition to complete history and physical
    - Relation to basal body temperature elevation to discover if it is painful ovulation.
    - *Labs:* Complete blood count (CBC), pregnancy test, STI (serotest for syphilis), urinalysis (UA), occult blood, blood culture.
    - *Imaging:* Abdominal, renal or vaginal US/CT/MRI, barium enema, bone scan.
    - Colonoscopy, cystoscopy or diagnostic laparoscopy if all results are inconclusive.
- **Acute pelvic pain**
  - *Causes requiring surgery:* Ruptured ovarian cyst (most common), adnexal torsion, tubo-ovarian abscess, ectopic pregnancy, appendicitis.
  - *Nonsurgical causes:* Abortion (spontaneous, threatened, incomplete), diverticulitis, UTI,

Inflammatory bowel disease (IBD), irritable bowel syndrome (IBS).
- Work-up in addition to complete history and physical.
  - *PID signs:* Cervical motion tenderness, adnexal and abdominal tenderness.
  - *Labs:* Pregnancy test, beta-hCG (serial assessment), CBC, UA.
  - Pelvic sonogram with possible need for diagnostic laparoscopy.

PELVIC INFLAMMATORY DISEASE

- Inflammation of the female upper genital tract (uterus, tubes, ovaries, ligaments) caused by ascending infection from the vagina and cervix. Common organisms: *Neisseria gonorrhoeae, Chlamydia, E. coli, Bacteroides*.
- Diagnosis
  - *Physical examination:* Abdominal, adnexal and cervical motion tenderness.
  - Fever, gram-positive stain, pelvic abscess, leukocytosis, purulent cervical discharge.
  - Laparoscopy is the gold standard for diagnosis, but is reserved for cases unresponsive to medical treatment.
- *Risk factors:* Multiple sexual partners, new sex partner(s), unprotected intercourse, concomitant history of sexually transmitted disease.
- *Criteria for hospitalization:* Pregnancy, peritonitis, gastrointestinal (GI) symptoms (nausea, vomiting), abscess (tubo-ovarian or pelvic), and uncertain diagnosis.

- Inpatient treatment
    - Cefotetan + Doxycycline (preferred for *Chlamydia*)
    - Clindamycin + Gentamicin (preferred for abscess)
- Outpatient treatment: Treat sexual partners also.
    - Ofloxacin + Metronidazole
    - Ceftriaxone + Doxycycline (preferred for *Chlamydia* (because of doxycycline).
- Differential of suspected PID
    - *GYN:* Ectopic pregnancy, hemorrhagic ovarian cyst or torsion, endometriosis.
    - *GI:* Appendicitis, cholecystitis, gastroenteritis, IBS
    - *Urinary:* Nephrolithiasis, UTI
    - *Psych:* Somatization

TOXIC SHOCK SYNDROME

- Toxic shock syndrome (TSS) is caused by the Toxic Shock Syndrome Toxin -1 (TSST-1) of *Staphylococcus aureus*.
    - Cases have been associated with menstruation and the use of super absorbent tampons.
    - *Half of cases are nonmenstrual:* Postsurgical, postpartum, burns, after sinusitis, enterocolitis or respiratory infections following influenza.
- *Criteria for TSS:* Three different organ systems involved or is there a fever >38.9°C
    - Mucus membranes, GI, liver, renal, skin, cardiac, muscular, hematologic, skin rash, CNS.
- Potential sites for *Staphylococcus aureus*
    - *Males:* Surgical wounds, trauma sites, nasal

- *Females:* Male sources plus retained tampon or contraception sponge.
- Management
  - Stabilize hemodynamics, replace volume and electrolytes.
  - Remove any foreign bodies, culture blood and wound sites.
  - IV Clindamycin inhibits protein synthesis, which stops toxin production (600 q8 hours) plus.
  - If MRSA for cell lysis—Vancomycin 20 mg/kg/dose q 8–12 hours (max 2g/dose).
  - If MSSA use the antistaph beta lactam Nafcillin 2g q4 hour.
  - If there is a known resistance to Clindamycin—use Linezolid 600 q 12 hours.

INCONTINENCE AND PELVIC ORGAN PROLAPSE

- *Stress:* Leakage of urine with a cough, sneeze, exercise, laugh and Valsalva.
- *Urge:* Incontinence on the way to the bathroom, leaking.
- *Overflow:* Continuous urine loss without urgency, post-void fullness.
  - *Q-tip test:* Urethral rotation at rest and with strain (30 degree is abnormal).
  - 24 hour voiding diary. Bladder retraining-use the restroom on schedule every 2–3 hours.
  - *Urge type:* Oxybutynin 2.5–5 mg TID; Imipramine 10–25 TID; Hyoscyamine 0.125–0.25 QID.

- *Overflow type:* Stop tricyclics, benzos, antispasmodics, antiparkinsonians, calcium blockers, etc.
- Pelvic floor relaxation is most commonly caused by childbirth. This can cause bowel or bladder incontinence, pain and infections.
  - Types include uterine, bladder (cystocele), rectal (rectocele), intestinal (enterocele).
- Uterine prolapse is graded on relation to introitus:
  - *Grade I:* Cervix halfway to introitus
  - *Grade II:* Cervix at the introitus
  - *Grade III:* Cervix outside the introitus
  - *Grade IV:* Entire uterus outside the introitus
- Management of urinary incontinence and all types of prolapse
  - *Medical:* Minor pelvic relaxation should practice Kegels to strengthen pelvic floor. Estrogen replacement may help in postmenopausal women. Pessaries elevate structures into their correct positions. Reduce coughing, reduce pm fluid intake.
  - *Surgical:* It is considered when medical management fails. Vaginal hysterectomy with a vaginal repair aims to repair the wall areas that are weak.

GESTATIONAL TROPHOBLASTIC DISEASE

- An occasional cause of first trimester bleeding caused by neoplasms arising from placental syncytio- or cytotrophoblast.
  - *Hydatidiform mole*

- *Complete mole:* Ultrasound shows multiple vesicular spaces without a fetus. Maternal ovum without DNA that is fertilized by sperm.
- *Partial:* Mole with fetal parts, with both maternal and paternal DNA.
- *Signs:* Uterus larger than dates, absent fetal heartbeat, higher than normal hCG levels, hyperemesis or thyrotoxicosis, ovarian enlargement from ovarian hyperstimulation, grape-like vesicles passing in second trimester.
  - *Invasive mole:* Mole that invades the myometrium; malignant form of GTD.
  - *Choriocarcinoma:* Epithelial tumor without villi, same treatment as metastatic moles.
- *Workup:* hCG > 100,000 mIU/mL, absence of fetal heartbeat, ultrasound findings and pathologic results.
- *Treatment:* Uterine D&C, followed by weekly hCGs for 2 months with strict contraception. If hCG rises, it is considered to be malignant (choriocarcinoma).
  - *Look for metastasis:* CXR, LFTs, CT brain, liver, lung and kidneys
  - Chemotherapy—Methotrexate or Actinomycin-D (until hCG levels normalize)
  - Or, total abdominal hysterectomy + chemotherapy (fewer cycles needed).

OVARIAN CYST MANAGEMENT

- Differential diagnosis of complex ovarian cysts:

- *GYN:* Endometriosis (endometrioma), ectopic pregnancy, ovarian cyst/neoplasm, suspected tubo-ovarian abscess, pelvic hematoma
- *GI:* Appendicitis, periappendiceal abscess, IBS.
- Concerning features in a complex cyst are: thick septations >3 mm, solid components with Doppler flow, excrescences, surrounding ascites
- *Premenopausal simple ovarian cyst*
  - *< 5 cm:* No follow-up needed
  - *5-10 cm:* Symptom management
  - *>10 cm:* Offer surgery
- *Premenopausal complex ovarian cyst*
  - *<5 cm:* No follow-up
  - *>5 cm:* Follow-up in 3 months and offer surgery if not resolved
  - If there are concerning features may offer surgery sooner and if smaller.
- *Postmenopausal simple ovarian cyst*
  - *<3 cm:* No follow-up
  - *3-10 cm:* Follow-up and if persists in 6 months, may offer surgery
  - *>10 cm:* Offer surgery
- *Postmenopausal complex ovarian cyst without concerning features*
  - *<5 cm:* Follow-up in 6 weeks, if unchanged follow at 3 months, 6 months, then yearly. If gains concerning features or grows, offer surgery
  - *>5 cm:* Offer surgery

- *Ovarian cysts in 2nd trimester pregnancy*
  - *Simple cyst of any size:* Conservative management
  - *Dermoid cyst without ascites:* Conservative management
  - *Complex mass >8 cm:* Offer surgery

CANCER SCREENING DON'TS

- Do not perform routine annual cervical cytology screening (Pap tests) in women 30–65 years of age.
  - In average risk women, annual cervical cytology screening has been shown to offer no advantage over screening performed at 3-year intervals.
  - However, a well-woman visit should occur annually for patients with their health care practitioner to discuss concerns and problems, and have appropriate screening with consideration of a pelvic examination.
- Do not treat patients who have mild dysplasia of less than two years in duration.
  - Mild dysplasia (cervical intraepithelial neoplasia [CIN 1]) is associated with the presence of the human papillomavirus (HPV), which does not require treatment in average risk women. Most women with CIN 1 on biopsy have a transient HPV infection that will usually clear in less than 12 months and, therefore, does not require treatment.
- Do not screen for ovarian cancer in asymptomatic women at average risk.
  - In population studies, there is only fair evidence that screening of asymptomatic women with serum CA-125

level and/or transvaginal (color Doppler) ultrasound can detect ovarian cancer at an earlier stage than it can be detected in the absence of screening. Because of the low prevalence of ovarian cancer and the invasive nature of the interventions following a positive screening test, the potential harms of screening outweigh the potential benefits.

CERVICAL DYSPLASIA CLASSIFICATION

- The Bethesda system or squamous intraepithelial lesion (SIL) is a cytological system which classifies individual cells from a Pap smear or liquid-based cytology according to the degree of cell abnormality. These break down into:
  - Atypical squamous cells of undetermined significance (ASCUS), used to identify cell abnormality which are not clearly dysplastic. This can be due to a variety of factors, including hormonal changes, yeast or other infections, medications, or other sources of inflammation. Reflex testing for HPV to triage patients according to the presence or absence of high-risk viral subtypes.
  - ASC-H (atypical squamous cells, favor dysplasia), a subtype of ASCUS, which identifies cells that are felt to be at higher risk for being dysplastic. These are usually followed with colposcopy and biopsy.
  - AGUS or AGCUS (atypical glandular cells of undetermined significance), a finding of atypical glandular cells. These patients should be evaluated

for endometrial or endocervical cancer. Low-grade squamous intraepithelial lesion (LSIL) usually corresponds to CIN I or mild dysplasia. These patients should undergo colposcopy.
- High-grade squamous intraepithelial lesion (HSIL), corresponds usually to CIN II or CIN III and these patients should be referred for colposcopy and biopsy.

GYNECOLOGIC CANCER

- *Uterine cancer:* Endometrial carcinoma is the most common gynecologic malignancy.
  - Caused by unopposed estrogen that hyperstimulates the endometrium.
  - Risk factors include obesity, hypertension, diabetes mellitus, nulliparity, late menopause and anovulatory conditions like polycystic ovarian syndrome.
  - Usually diagnosed with endometrial biopsy and/or D&C.
  - Treated with hysterectomy and salpingo-oopherectomy. Postsurgical pathology determines need for radiation or chemotherapy.
- *Cervical cancer* is screened for by the Pap smear
  - "Treatment and prognosis of the cervical cancer depends on the stage and type of the cancer, age of the patient, history and desire to preserve fertility".
  - *Invasive cervical cancer:* Treated with hysterectomy plus radiation and chemotherapy.
- *Ovarian cancer:* Complex mass usually detected by ultrasound; surgery is the initial treatment of choice (tumor debulking or cytoreduction), followed by chemotherapy.

- *Vulvar carcinoma* is rare, and its most common symptom is vulvar itching
  - Most common type is squamous cell. Biopsy all vulvar lesions. Therapy is usually surgical. Radiation, chemotherapy and biologic therapy can also be used.

CERVICAL CANCER FIGO STAGING

- *Stage 0:* Carcinoma *in situ* (CIS); CIN III. Also called premalignant or precancerous.
- *Stage I:* Cancer in the cervix only
  - Ia—Invasion of the cervical tissues can only be seen with a microscope.
  - Ia1—Stromal invasion not more than 3.0 mm and extension not more than 7.0 mm.
  - Ia2—Stromal invasion more than 3.0 mm but not more than 5.0 mm and extension not more than 7.0 mm.
  - Ib—Lesions wider than 7 mm or deeper than 5 mm, or that can be seen without a microscope.
  - Ib1—Lesions less than 4.0 cm.
  - Ib2—Lesions more than 4.0 cm.
- *Stage II:* Cancer extends beyond the cervix, but not as far as the pelvic wall or the lower third of the vagina.
  - IIa—Extends to upper part of the vagina, but not to the surrounding tissues (parametria).
  - IIb—Extends to the parametrial tissues (but not to the pelvic wall).
- *Stage III:* The cancer has extended to the lower third of the vagina or to the pelvic wall.

- IIIa—The cancer has spread to the lower third of the vagina, but nowhere else.
- IIIb—The cancer has spread to the pelvic wall or caused hydronephrosis.
- *Stage IV:* Cancer has spread to the bladder, rectum, or outside the pelvis.
  - IVa—Spread to the rectum or bladder.
  - IVb—Metastasis to distant organs such as the lungs or liver.

ENDOMETRIAL CANCER FIGO STAGING

- *Stage I:* Cancer remains in the body of the uterus.
  - Ia—Cancer is in the endometrium only.
  - Ib—Cancer has invaded less than half of the thickness of the myometrium.
  - Ic—Cancer has extended to more than half of the thickness of the myometrium.
- *Stage II:* Cancer has extended to the cervix.
  - IIa—The cancer is only in the glands of the endocervix.
  - IIb—The cancer has invaded deeper into the cervical stromal.
- *Stage III:* Cancer has spread beyond the uterus.
  - IIIa—Invasion of the serosa and/or adnexa and/or positive pelvic washings.
  - IIIb—Spread to the vagina.
  - IIIc—Spread to the pelvic and/or para-aortic lymph nodes.
- *Stage IV:* More distant spread of the cancer.
  - IVa—To the mucosa of the rectum or bladder.

- IVb—Distant metastases including intra-abdominal and/or inguinal lymph nodes.

OVARIAN CANCER FIGO STAGING

- *Stage I:* Ovarian cancer remains in the ovaries.
    - Ia—Cancer is in one ovary, with the capsule intact and no tumor visible on the surface, and no positive pelvic washings.
    - Ib—Cancer is in both ovaries, but otherwise as above.
    - Ic—Stage Ia or Ib, but cancer is either visible on the outside of the ovary or the capsule has burst or there is ascites with malignant cells or positive peritoneal washings.
- *Stage II:* Cancer has spread inside the pelvis, but not beyond.
    - IIa—Tumor has spread to the tubes and/or the uterus.
    - IIb—Tumor has spread to other parts of the pelvis, but no cancer cells are found in ascites or peritoneal washings.
    - IIc—Stage IIa or IIb, but tumor is either visible on the outside of the ovary or the capsule has burst or there is ascites with malignant cells or positive peritoneal washings.
- *Stage III:* Cancer is found on the surfaces of abdominal organs and/or in nearby lymph nodes.
    - IIIa—Microscopic seeding of abdominal peritoneal surfaces.
    - IIIb—Abdominal implants smaller than 2 cm.

- IIIc—Abdominal implants larger than 2 cm and/or positive retroperitoneal or inguinal nodes.
- *Stage IV:* Distant metastases; pleural effusion with positive cytology; parenchymal liver metastasis.

VAGINAL AND VULVAR CANCER FIGO STAGING

Vaginal Cancer Staging

- *Stage 0:* Carcinoma *in situ*, VAIN 3, severe vaginal dysplasia. Not malignant.
- *Stage I:* Cancer is limited to the wall of the vagina.
- *Stage II:* Cancer has extended through the vaginal wall, into the parametrium, but not as far as the wall of the pelvis.
- *Stage III:* Cancer has extended to the pelvic wall and/or to the local lymph nodes.
- *Stage IV:* Cancer has invaded the bladder or rectum and/or spread outside the pelvis.
    - IVa—Tumor has spread to the inside of the bladder or rectum.
    - IVb—Tumor has spread outside the pelvic area.

Vulvar Cancer Staging

- *Stage 0:* Carcinoma *in situ*, VIN 3, severe vulvar dysplasia. This is not malignant.
- *Stage I:* Confined to vulva or perineum, tumor 2 cm or less.
    - Ia—Less than 1 mm of stromal invasion.
    - Ib—More than 1 mm of stromal invasion.
- *Stage II:* Cancer is confined to the vulva and/or perineum and larger than 2 cm. Nodes are negative.

- *Stage III:* Cancer has spread to the lower urethra or vagina or anus and/or local lymph nodes on one side only.
  - IVa—Cancer has spread to the upper urethra or bladder or rectum or local lymph nodes on both sides.
  - IVb—Cancer has spread to the pelvic lymph nodes and/or sites more distant.

BIBLIOGRAPHY

ACOG Committee on Practice Bulletins—Gynecology. ACOG Practice Bulletin No. 85: Pelvic organ prolapse. Obstet Gynecol 2007;110(3):717-29.

Altman D, Falconer C, Cnattingius S, Granath F. Pelvic organ prolapse surgery following hysterectomy on benign indications. Am J Obstet Gynecol 2008;198(5):572.e1-6.

American College of Obstetricians and Gynecologists Women's Health Care Physicians. Executive summary. Hormone therapy. Obstet Gynecol 2004;104:1S.

American College of Obstetricians and Gynecologists. ACOG Practice Bulletin. Management of adnexal masses. Obstet Gynecol 2007;110:201.

American Joint Committee on Cancer. Corpus Uteri. In: AJCC Staging Manual, 7th edn, Springer, New York; 2010. p.403.

Balleyguier C, Sala E, Da Cunha T, et al. Staging of uterine cervical cancer with MRI: guidelines of the European Society of Urogenital Radiology. Eur Radiol 2011;21:1102.

Beddy P, Moyle P, Kataoka M, et al. Evaluation of depth of myometrial invasion and overall staging in endometrial cancer: comparison of diffusion-weighted and dynamic contrast-enhanced MR imaging. Radiology 2012;262:530.

Benedet JL, Bender H, Jones H 3rd, et al. FIGO staging classifications and clinical practice guidelines in the management of gynecologic cancers. FIGO Committee on Gynecologic Oncology. Int J Gynaecol Obstet 2000;70:209.

Berghella V, Baxter JK, Chauhan SP. Evidence-based labor and delivery management. Am J Obstet Gynecol 2008;199:445.

Buys SS, Partridge E, Greene MH, et al. Ovarian cancer screening in the Prostate, Lung, Colorectal and Ovarian (PLCO) cancer screening trial: findings from the initial screen of a randomized trial. Am J Obstet Gynecol 2005;193:1630.

Cervix Uteri. In: Edge SB, Byrd DR, Compton CC, et al (Eds). American Joint Committee on Cancer Staging Manual, 7th edn, Springer, New York; 2010. p.395.

Clarke A, Black N, Rowe P, et al. Indications for and outcome of total abdominal hysterectomy for benign disease: a prospective cohort study. Br J Obstet Gynaecol 1995;102:611.

Clemons JL, Aguilar VC, Tillinghast TA, Jackson ND, Myers DL. Patient satisfaction and changes in prolapse and urinary symptoms in women who were fitted successfully with a pessary for pelvic organ prolapse. Am J Obstet Gynecol 2004;190(4):1025-29.

Committee on Practice Bulletins—Gynecology. Practice bulletin no. 128: diagnosis of abnormal uterine bleeding in reproductive-aged women. Obstet Gynecol 2012;120:197.

Dasharathy SS, Mumford SL, Pollack AZ, et al. Menstrual bleeding patterns among regularly menstruating women. Am J Epidemiol 2012;175:536.

de la Torre SH, Mandel L, Goff BA. Evaluation of postoperative fever: usefulness and cost-effectiveness of routine workup. Am J Obstet Gynecol 2003;188:1642.

Gillespie AM, Lidbury EA, Tidy JA, Hancock BW. The clinical presentation, treatment, and outcome of patients diagnosed with possible ectopic molar gestation. Int J Gynecol Cancer 2004;14:366.

Hernandez E, for the American College of Obstetricians and Gynecologists. Management of endometrial cancer. ACOG Practice Bulletin no. 65. Obstet Gynecol 2005;106(2):413-25.

Hoskins WJ, Perez CA, Young RC, Barakat RR, Markman M, Randall ME (Eds). Principles and Practice of Gynecologic Oncology, 4th edn. Philadelphia, Pa.: Lippincott Williams & Wilkins; 2000. pp.823-72.

Hurskainen R, Aalto AM, Teperi J, et al. Psychosocial and other characteristics of women complaining of menorrhagia, with and without actual increased menstrual blood loss. BJOG 2001;108:281.

Jacobs I. Genetic, biochemical, and multimodal approaches to screening for ovarian cancer. Gynecol Oncol 1994;55:S22.

Joste N. Overview of the cytology laboratory: specimen processing through diagnosis. Obstet Gynecol Clin North Am 2008;35:549.

Kakuno Y, Amino N, Kanoh M, et al. Menstrual disturbances in various thyroid diseases. Endocr J 2010;57:1017.

Kupesic Plavsic S, et al. Abnormal Genital Tract Bleeding. Video Atlas of Clinical Skills in Ob Gyn, Jaypee Brothers Medical Publisher; 2012.

Kupesic Plavsic S, et al. Abnormal Menstrual Cycle. Video Atlas of Clinical Skills in Ob Gyn, Jaypee Brothers Medical Publisher; 2012.

Kupesic Plavsic S, et al. Pelvic Masses and Pelvic Pain. Video Atlas of Clinical Skills in Ob Gyn, Jaypee Brothers Medical Publisher; 2012.

Kupesic Plavsic S, et al. Vaginal Discharge, STD and PID. Video Atlas of Clinical Skills in Ob Gyn, Jaypee Brothers Medical Publisher; 2012.

Lamvu G, Steege JF. The anatomy and neurophysiology of pelvic pain. J Minim Invasive Gynecol 2006;13:516.

Lanham M, Morgan H. University of Michigan OB-Gyn Survival Guide, 2011.

Mason A, Goldacre M, Meddings D, Woolfson J. Use of case fatality and readmission measures to compare hospital performance in gynaecology. BJOG 2006;113:695.

Matteson KA, Boardman LA, Munro MG, Clark MA. Abnormal uterine bleeding: a review of patient-based outcome measures. Fertil Steril 2009;92:205.

McDonald JM, Modesitt SC. The incidental postmenopausal adnexal mass. Clin Obstet Gynecol 2006;49:506.

Parsonnet J, Hansmann MA, Delaney ML, et al. Prevalence of toxic shock syndrome toxin 1-producing *Staphylococcus aureus* and the presence of antibodies to this superantigen in menstruating women. J Clin Microbiol 2005;43:4628.

Pavlik EJ, Ueland FR, Miller RW, et al. Frequency and disposition of ovarian abnormalities followed with serial transvaginal ultrasonography. Obstet Gynecol 2013;122:210.

Pecorelli S. Revised FIGO staging for carcinoma of the vulva, cervix, and endometrium. Int J Gynaecol Obstet. 2009;105:103.

Price J, Farmer G, Harris J, et al. Attitudes of women with chronic pelvic pain to the gynaecological consultation: a qualitative study. BJOG 2006;113:446.

Schlievert PM. Role of superantigens in human disease. J Infect Dis 1993;167:997.

Shifren JL, Schiff I. Role of hormone therapy in the management of menopause. Obstet Gynecol 2010;115:839.

Singh N, Arif S. Histopathologic parameters of prognosis in cervical cancer—a review. Int J Gynecol Cancer 2004;14:741.

Smith HO. Gestational trophoblastic disease epidemiology and trends. Clin Obstet Gynecol 2003;46:541.

Solomon D, Davey D, Kurman R, et al. The 2001 Bethesda System: terminology for reporting results of cervical cytology. JAMA 2002;287:2114.

Soper DE. Pelvic inflammatory disease. Obstet Gynecol 2010;116:419.

Soper JT. Gestational trophoblastic disease. Obstet Gynecol 2006;108:176.

Stevens DL, Wallace RJ, Hamilton SM, Bryant AE. Successful treatment of staphylococcal toxic shock syndrome with linezolid: a case report and *in vitro* evaluation of the production of toxic shock syndrome toxin type 1 in the presence of antibiotics. Clin Infect Dis 2006;42:729.

Stewart FH, Harper CC, Ellertson CE, et al. Clinical breast and pelvic examination requirements for hormonal contraception: Current practice vs evidence. JAMA 2001;285:2232.

Thurston RC, Joffe H. Vasomotor symptoms and menopause: findings from the Study of Women's Health across the Nation. Obstet Gynecol Clin North Am 2011;38:489.

Todo Y, Sakuragi N, Nishida R, et al. Combined use of magnetic resonance imaging, CA 125 assay, histologic type, and histologic grade in the prediction of lymph node metastasis in endometrial carcinoma. Am J Obstet Gynecol 2003;188:1265.

U.S. Preventive Services Task Force. Am Fam Physician 2005;71(4):759-62.

U.S. Preventive Services Task Force. Screening for ovarian cancer: recommendation statement. 2012;157(12):900-4.

University Hospitals Case Medical Center, MacDonald Women's Hospital. Resident's Manual, 2007.

Warner PE, Critchley HO, Lumsden MA, et al. Menorrhagia I: measured blood loss, clinical features, and outcome in women with heavy periods: a survey with follow-up data. Am J Obstet Gynecol 2004;190:1216.

Waxman AG, Chelmow D, Darragh TM, et al. Revised terminology for cervical histopathology and its implications for management of high-grade squamous intraepithelial lesions of the cervix. Obstet Gynecol 2012;120:1465.

Zeger W, Holt K. Gynecologic infections. Emerg Med Clin North Am 2003;21:631.

Index

A

Abdomen 11
Abdominal disorders 45
Abdominal wall 109
Abortion 60, 73, 125
    incomplete 125
    methods 61
    missed 53
    spontaneous 53, 125
    threatened 53, 125
Adrenal gland 24
Allergies 73
Amenorrhea 121
Aminoglycosides 63
Amniocentesis 15
Amnioinfusion 21
Amniotic fluid 17
    index 17
Amphetamines 110
Androgens 63
Anemia 19
Anesthesia 118
    epidural 81
Angiotensin-converting enzyme inhibitors 64
Antibiotics 13, 63
Anticonvulsant therapy 44
Anticonvulsive therapy
    magnesium sulfate 48
Antiretroviral therapy 41
Appendicitis 45
Apt test 54
Atypical glandular cells 133
Atypical squamous cells 133

B

Bethesda system 133
Bishop's score 5, 80
Blood pressure
    diastolic 27
    systolic 48
Blood urea nitrogen 47
Bradycardia 19
Braxton Hicks contractions 76
Breast milk, stages of 111
Breastfeeding 110
Breech 101
    complete 101
    frank 101
    incomplete 101
    position, types of 101
    vaginal delivery, trial of 101
Bromocriptine 110

C

Calcium channel blockers 93
Cancer FIGO staging
    cervical 135

    endometrial 136
    vaginal and vulvar 138
Cancer
    cervical 124, 134
    ecologic 134
    ovarian 134
    uterine 134
    vulvar 124
Carbamazepine 62
Central nervous system 29, 46
Cephalopelvic disproportion 96, 97
Cerebral blood flow, loss of
    regulation of 48
Cervical dysplasia classification 133
Cervical intraepithelial neoplasia 132
Chills 73
Chlamydia 55
Cholecystitis 45
Choriocarcinoma 130
Chorionic villus sampling 15
Cocaine 110
Complete blood cell 5
Constipation 25, 73
Contraception 108
Contraction stress test 17
Convulsions, control of 48
Cordocentesis 15
Cyclophosphamide 110
Cyclosporine 110
Cytomegalovirus infection 110

D

Deep tendon reflexes 3
Deep vein thrombosis 50
Dehydration 19
Dermoid cyst 132
Diabetes mellitus, gestational 40
Diarrhea 73
Digital cervical examination 79
Disseminated intravascular
    coagulation 61
Doppler fetal heart tones 11
Down's syndrome 6
Doxorubicin 110
Dysfunctional uterine
    bleeding 121
Dysmenorrhea 121
Dyspareunia 123
Dysplasia, favor 133
Dysuria 73

E

Eclampsia 46, 48
Endometriosis 118
Endometrium 109
Epilepsy 44
Episiotomy 106
    infection 111
Ergotamine 110
Erythrocyte sedimentation
    rate 27
Estimated date of delivery (EDD) 5
Estrogen-secreting tumor 124

F

Family planning 108
Ferning test 77, 78

Fertility 118
Fetal
    abdominal measurements 16
    assessment 13
    death 46
    demise 59
    distress, signs of 3
    growth restriction 46
    heart tone 5
    movement 17, 19
    tachycardia 19
    ultrasound testing 16
Fever 73
First trimester bleeding 52
Flexion 83
Fluorescent *in situ* hybridization (FISH) 16
Folic acid derivatives 62
Forceps delivery 90
Fundal height 11

G

Gallbladder 25
Gastrointestinal system 25
Genital neoplasm 118
Genitourinary system 28
Glucagon 23
Glucose challenge screening test 40
Gonorrhea 55

H

Heart failure 46
Heart sounds 26
HELLP syndrome 46, 49
Hematuria 73
Hemolysis 49
Hemorrhage, cerebral 46
Hemostasis 106
Hepatitis
    B infection 110
    C virus 5
Herpes simplex virus 110
High-density lipoprotein 22
High-grade squamous intraepithelial lesion 134
HIV infection 110
Hormonal replacement therapy 123
Hot flashes 123
Human chorionic gonadotropin 23
Human papillomavirus 132
Human placental lactogen 23
Hypermenorrhea 121
Hyperplasia, endometrial 124
Hypertension
    chronic 57
    gestational 46, 47
Hyperthermia 19
Hypomenorrhea 121
Hypothyroidism 43

I

Imipramine 62
In vitro fertilization 58
Inflammatory bowel disease 126
Intrapartum fetal monitoring 18
Intrauterine growth restriction 2, 16, 42
Invasive mole 130
Irritable bowel syndrome 126

J

Joint pain, swelling 73

K

Kick counts 17
Kleihauer-Betke test 54

L

Labor
    abnormal 88
    dystocia 96
    induction 88
    movements 83
    pain control 80
    progress, vaginal delivery notes 72
    recognize signs of 38
    stages of 81
Leiomyoma 125
Leopold maneuvers 13, 101
Leukocytosis 110
Lithium 110
Liver 25
    function tests 47
Lochia alba 109
Lochia rubra 109
Lochia serosa 109
Low back pain 38
Low density lipoprotein 22
Low grade squamous intraepithelial lesion 134
Low transverse cesarean section 89
Lower urinary tract atrophy 123
Lower uterine segment 109
Lumbar block 81

M

Macrosomia 98
Magnesium sulfate 49
Marijuana 110
Mastitis 112
    endemic 112
Maternal fetal medicine 2
Maternal fever 19
Maternal serum alpha-fetoprotein 6
McBurney's point 45
McRoberts maneuver 100
Melanocyte-stimulating hormone 29
Membranes
    premature rupture of 95
    preterm premature rupture of 95
    prolonged rupture of 78
    rupture of 38, 77
Menometrorrhagia 121
Menopause 123
Menorrhagia 121
Methotrexate 110
Metrorrhagia 121
Mifepristone 61
Mild dysplasia 132
Mole
    complete 130
    hydatidiform 129

N

Naegele's rule 7
Naloxone hydrochloride 81

Nausea 38, 73
Neisseria gonorrhoeae 126
Neoplasia 125
Nicotine 110
Nifedipine 48, 93
Nitrazine test 77, 79
Non-stress test 17, 47

O

Oligomenorrhea 121
Osteoporosis 123
Ovarian cyst 131, 132
    management 130
Ovulatory dub 122
Oxytocin 89

P

Pain 120
    abdominal 73
    medications 63
    relief 81
Parathyroid glands 23
Partial placenta previa 56
Pelvic floor relaxation 129
Pelvic infections 117
Pelvic inflammatory disease 125, 126
Pelvic pain 123
    acute 125
    chronic 125
Peripartum cardiomyopathy 51
Peritonitis 126
Phencyclidine 110
Placenta accreta 97
Placenta increta 98
Placenta percreta 98
Placenta previa 56, 122
Placental abruption 46, 57
Platelet count 47
Polymenorrhea 120
Pool test 77
Postcoital bleeding 122
Posterior shoulder delivery 100
Postmenopausal simple ovarian cyst 131
Postmenopausal vaginal bleeding 124
Postpartum depression 112
Postpartum hemorrhage 98
Postpartum psychosis 113
Postpartum thyroiditis 44
Pre-eclampsia 46, 47
Pregnancy
    acute abdomen in 45
    acute fatty liver of 50
    complications 37
    ectopic 55
    HIV in 41
    termination of 60
Prostaglandins 89
Protraction disorders 96
Pulmonary edema 3
Pulmonary embolism 51

Q

Q-tip test 128
Quad test, combined 6

R

Reflux esophagitis 25
Renal disorders 45
Renal failure 3
Renal system 29
Respiratory depression 3
Respiratory distress syndrome 96
Rhesus alloimmunization 9

S

Sheehan syndrome 44
Shoulder dystocia 100
Skin 29
Squamous intraepithelial lesion 133
Staphylococcus aureus 112, 127
Sterile vaginal exam 39, 74
Stress 128
Surgery, abdominal 120
Swelling 38
Systolic dysfunction, symptoms of 52

T

Tachycardia 19
Tay-Sachs disease 60
Thrombosis 50
Thyroid gland 23
Toxic shock syndrome 127
Trophoblastic disease,
     gestational 129

U

Uric acid 47
Urinary tract 109
Uterine bleeding 120
    abnormal 121
Uterine inversion 98
Uterine rupture 58
Uterus 109

V

Vaginal atrophy 123, 124
Vaginal bleeding 38
    premenopausal 124
Vaginal cancer staging 138
Vaginal delivery 75
Vaginal discharge, abnormal 73
Vaginal surgery 120
Valproic acid 62
Vasa previa 58
Vitamin A 62
    Vomiting 38, 73
    Vulvar carcinoma 135

W

White blood cells 27
Woods Corkscrew maneuver 100
Worsening blood pressure 3
Wright's stain 54

Z

Zavanelli maneuver 100